Illustrated Signs in Clinical Medicine

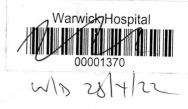

Illustrated Signs in Clinical Medicine

K C McHardy MD FRCPE
Consultant Physician and Postgraduate Tutor,
Aberdeen Royal Infirmary, UK

K P Duguid FRPS
Director, Department of Medical Illustration,
University of Aberdeen, UK

M J Jamieson MRCP
Assistant Professor, Division of Clinical Pharmacology,
University of Texas Health Science Center, San Antonio, USA

J C Petrie CBE FRCP FRCPE FRCPI FFPM
Professor and Head of Department of Medicine and Therapeutics,
University of Aberdeen, UK

H M A Towler MRCP FRCSE
Consultant, Department of Ophthalmology,
Whipps Cross Hospital, London, UK

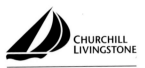

CHURCHILL
LIVINGSTONE

EDINBURGH LONDON MADRID MELBOURNE NEW YORK
SAN FRANCISCO AND TOKYO 1997

CHURCHILL LIVINGSTONE
Medical Division of Pearson Professional Limited

Distributed in the United States of America by Churchill
Livingstone Inc., 650 Avenue of the Americas, New York,
N.Y. 10011, and by associated companies, branches and
representatives throughout the world.

Text © Pearson Professional Limited 1997
Illustrations © Grampian Health Board 1990

First published 1997
Standard Edition ISBN 0 443 05545 9

International Edition first published 1997
International Edition ISBN 0 443 05617 X

British Library Cataloguing in Publication Data
A catalogue record for this book is available from the British
Library.

Library of Congress Cataloging in Publication Data
A catalog record for this book is available from the Library
of Congress.

Medical knowledge is constantly changing. As new
information becomes available, changes in treatment,
procedures, equipment and the use of drugs become
necessary. The authors and the publishers have, as far as it
is possible, taken care to ensure that the information given
in this text is accurate and up to date. However, readers are
strongly advised to confirm that the information, especially
with regard to drug usage, complies with current legislation
and standards of practice.

Produced by Longman Asia Limited, Hong Kong
SWT/01

Preface

This book contains over four hundred colour images of external and ocular physical signs selected by experienced medical teachers and illustrators covering an extensive range of clinical medicine. Originally published as an illustrated vocabulary (*Essential Clinical Signs*, 1990) this new publication has been modified in response to readers' requests for the addition of explanatory notes on each physical sign. Relating to appearance, aetiology and associated symptoms or signs, the new text greatly enhances the educational value of the illustrative material for everyone interested in health care. The quantity of text has however been limited for this remains essentially a picture book aiming to illustrate clinical medicine in a way which will encourage understanding of the significance, and aid subsequent recognition, of common or classical physical signs in medical practice.

We hope that the reader finds studying this annotated collection of images enjoyable, and goes on to find successful identification and recognition of physical signs 'in the field' even more rewarding.

KCMcH
Aberdeen, 1997

Acknowledgements

We would like to acknowledge the cooperation of the following colleagues in contributing material for this book:

Dr N Bruce Bennett; Miss F M Bennett; Dr P D Bewsher; Mr C T Blaicklock; Dr J Broom; Dr P W Brunt; Mr P B Clarke; Dr Gaynor Cole; Dr Audrey A Dawson; Professor A S Douglas; Dr J G Douglas; Dr A W Downie; Dr C J Eastmond; Dr Neil Edward; Mr J Engeset; Mr O M Fenton; Professor J V Forrester; Dr J A R Friend; Mr W H H Garvie; Mr Frank Green; Professor R L Himsworth; Dr A W Hutcheon; Mr C Hutchinson; Dr T A Jeffers; Dr A W Johnston; Mr R Keenan; Dr A C F Kenmure; Dr J S Legge; Dr R A Main; Mr K L G Mills; Dr N A G Mowat; Mr I F K Muir; Dr Lilian E Murchison; Mr W J Newlands; Dr D W M Pearson; Dr J Petersen; Dr J M Rawles; Mr P K Ray; Mr C R W Rayner; Dr D M Reid; Dr J A N Rennie; Professor D S Short; Dr C C Smith; Dr L Stankler; Professor J M Stowers; Dr J Webster; Dr Marion I White; Dr M J Williams; Mr G G Youngson.

We wish also to thank the patients who gave permission for their photographs to be reproduced here; general practices, the Primary Care Division and the Medical Records Department of Grampian Health Board for their help in tracing patients; and the staff of the Department of Medical Illustration of the University of Aberdeen. We are grateful to Moira Davidson for secretarial assistance and acknowledge Dr T M MacDonald and Mrs G Chessell for the contribution they made to the previously published *Essential Clinical Signs*.

Contents

1 Head and neck

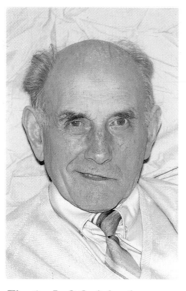

**Fig. 1a Left facial palsy –
upper motor neurone lesion**

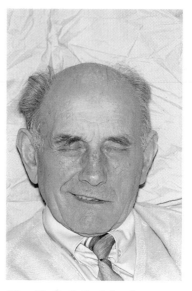

**Fig. 1b Left facial palsy –
eye closure**

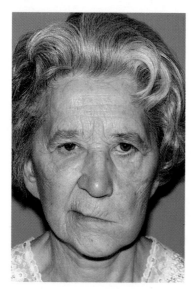

**Fig. 1c Left facial palsy –
lower motor neurone lesion**

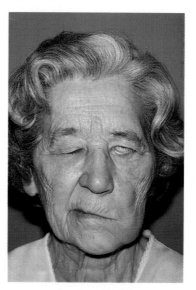

**Fig. 1d Left facial palsy –
incomplete eye closure**

Figure 1a–d Facial asymmetry with loss of the nasolabial fold on the affected side indicates facial nerve palsy. An upper motor neurone lesion (**Fig. 1a**), usually due to cerebrovascular disease, causes weakness of the lower part of the face only. Forehead movements and eye closure (**Fig. 1b**) are preserved because of bilateral cortical motor representation of the upper face. A lower motor neurone lesion (**Fig. 1c**), most commonly due to Bell's palsy, leads to weakness of the whole side of the face. Note incomplete eye closure (Bell's sign) which can leave the cornea exposed (**Fig. 1d**).

Fig. 2a Jaundice

Fig. 2b Jaundice

Fig. 2c Jaundice

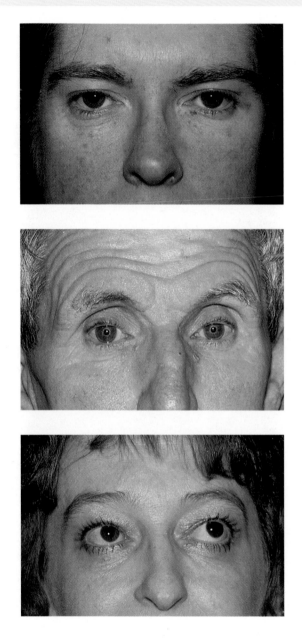

Figure 2a–c Jaundice is due to accumulation of circulating bile pigment deposits in connective tissues. Natural differences in skin tone may sometimes make assessment difficult. Inspection of normally white sclerae for yellow discoloration can be helpful. The threshold for detection of jaundice, or icterus, is at a serum bilirubin concentration of approximately 35 µmol/L. There are many causes and, while it may result from increased rates of haemolysis, e.g. autoimmune haemolytic anaemia, it is more often seen with intrinsic hepatic disease. This might be viral hepatitis, metastatic carcinoma, primary biliary cirrhosis, chronic active hepatitis or drug allergy. Alternatively, the cause may be biliary obstruction due to gall stones or pancreatic tumour, for example.

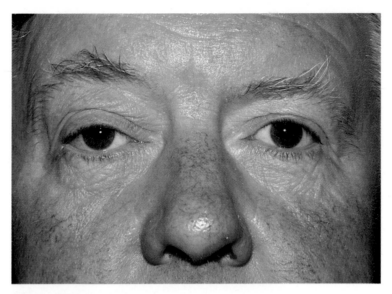

Fig. 3 Telangiectasia

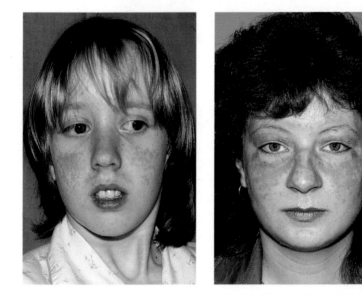

Fig. 4a Butterfly rash

Fig. 4b Butterfly rash

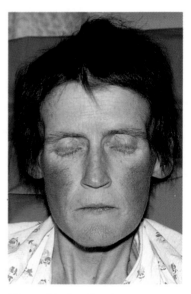

Fig. 5 Malar flush

Figure 3 Telangiectases are dilated skin capillaries, which are often a normal finding on the face, especially with increasing age.

Figure 4a–b Butterfly rash is a term used to describe the distribution of a rash where the nose represents the butterfly's body and the cheeks its wings. A blotchy rash in this distribution is a feature of systemic lupus erythematosus.

Figure 5 Malar flush is a diffuse dusky discoloration, sometimes with a telangiectatic component, occurring over the cheeks but typically sparing the nose. It may be associated with mitral valve stenosis, particularly when pulmonary hypertension has developed.

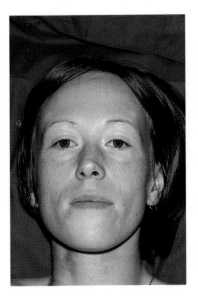

Fig. 6 Vitiligo

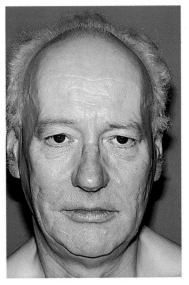

Fig. 7 Pallor

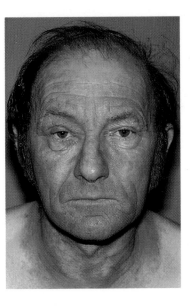

Fig. 8 Photosensitive rash

Figure 6 Vitiligo is dermal depigmentation. It occurs less frequently on the face than on the hands and may be associated with a predisposition to organ-specific autoimmune disease, such as Addison's disease, Hashimoto's thyroiditis and insulin-dependent diabetes mellitus.

Figure 7 Facial pallor is a clue to underlying anaemia, but it may occur due to peripheral vasoconstriction and may also be a natural variant (especially in red-haired Caucasians).

Figure 8 The distribution of a photosensitive rash, confined to light-exposed areas, is the main clue to the nature of this condition. The commonest aetiology is over-exposure to sunlight. Rarer causes include drug-dependent photosensitivity, systemic lupus erythematosus and porphyria.

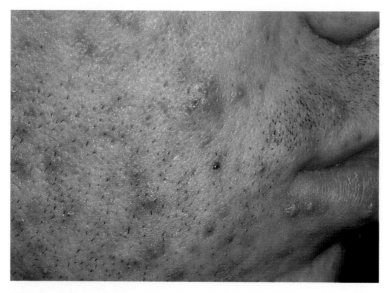

Fig. 9a Acne vulgaris

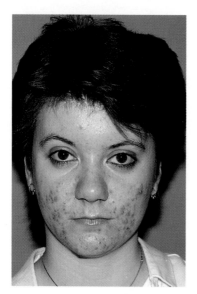

Fig. 9b Acne vulgaris

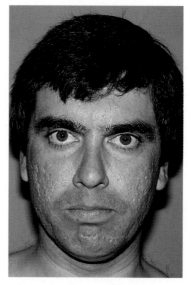

Fig. 9c Acne scarring

Figure 9a–c Acne vulgaris is a common skin condition particularly affecting adolescents and young adults (**Fig. 9a–b**). Its features include comedones (blackheads), papules, pustules and scabs, and it may lead to patchy dermal scarring (pock marks) (**Fig. 9c**).

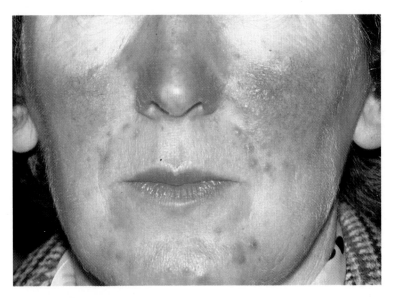

Fig. 10a Rosacea

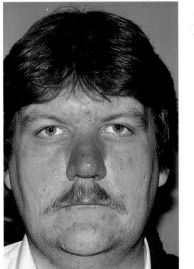

Fig. 10b Rosacea

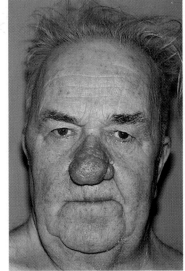

Fig. 11 Rhinophyma

Figure 10a–b Rosacea occurs over the face and features erythema, papules, pustules and sometimes telangiectases. Comedones are not a feature of this condition, which usually occurs after adolescence.

Figure 11 A late complication is hypertrophy of the nasal skin, or rhinophyma.

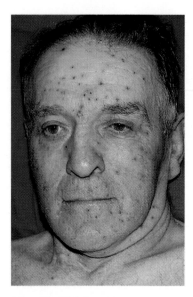

Fig. 12 Chickenpox

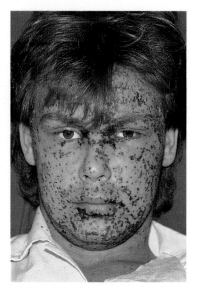

Fig. 13 Kaposi's
varicelliform eruption

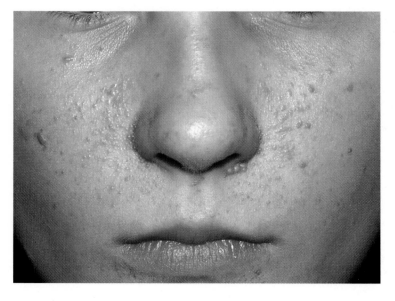

Fig. 14 Adenoma sebaceum

Figure 12 Several viral illnesses can cause skin lesions that go through the sequence: macule, papule, vesicle, pustule, scab. Chickenpox (commonest in children) has a predominantly peripheral distribution and lesions at different stages may be present simultaneously. In adults suffering from chickenpox (illustrated here), underlying immune deficiency disorders should be considered.

Figure 13 Kaposi's varicelliform eruption (eczema herpeticum) is a severe vesicular eruption normally due to *Herpes Simplex Virus (type I)* infection occurring on a background of a pre-existing skin disorder, most commonly atopic eczema.

Figure 14 Adenoma sebaceum consists of small fibromatous papules most commonly around the nose. This is one feature of epiloia (tuberous sclerosis).

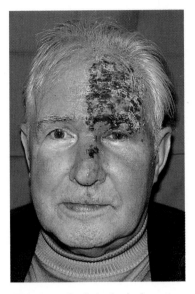

Fig. 15a Ophthalmic herpes zoster

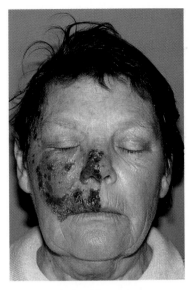

Fig. 15b Maxillary herpes zoster

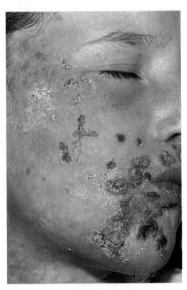

Fig. 15c Mandibular herpes zoster

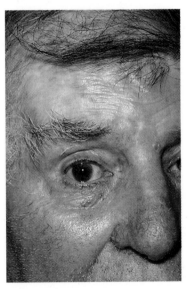

Fig. 15d Post-herpetic scarring

Figure 15a–d *Herpes Zoster Virus* causes painful vesiculation in a dermatomal distribution. On the face this typically affects one division of the trigeminal nerve. Note that the ophthalmic variant (**Fig. 15a**) can be associated with corneal disease and can extend on to the nose (nasociliary branch of ophthalmic division of trigeminal nerve). Maxillary (**Fig. 15b**) and mandibular disease (**Fig. 15c**) will also affect the corresponding intraoral area (see **Fig. 68**). Post-herpetic scarring (**Fig. 15d**) can leave irregular depigmentation in a dermatomal distribution.

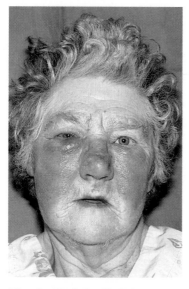

Fig. 16 Facial cellulitis

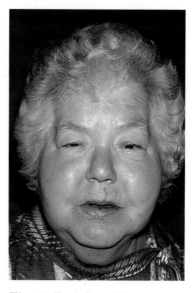

Fig. 17 Facial swelling

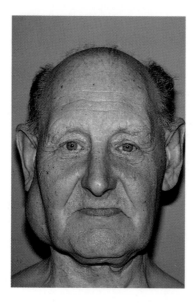

Fig. 18a Parotid swelling

Figure 16 Cellulitis, or soft-tissue infection, often affects the face. It is typically caused by *Streptococcal* infection and the dermal oedema and erythema may have a well-demarcated, even 'stepped', edge. The term erysipelas is sometimes used to describe this condition.

Figure 17 Facial swelling can be non-inflammatory, e.g. in hypoalbuminaemic states or right-sided cardiac failure. Superior vena cava obstruction would typically produce some discoloured engorged vessels in the neck or upper chest (see **Fig. 146**). Swelling of the lax tissues around the eyes distinguishes this appearance from the fatty deposition of Cushing's moon face (**Fig. 27a–b**).

Figure 18a–b Local swelling can occur around the face, e.g. in the parotid gland (**Fig. 18a**) or below the angle of the jaw at the anterior margin of sternomastoid as in a branchial cyst (**Fig. 18b**).

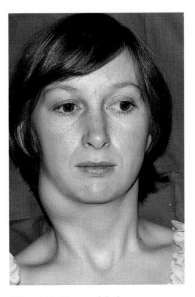

Fig. 18b Branchial cyst

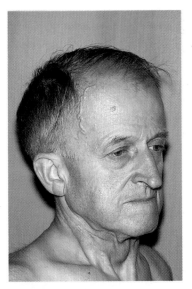

Fig. 19 Pagetic skull

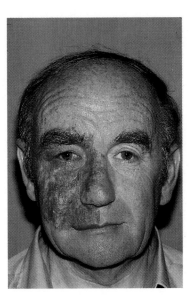

Fig. 20 Cavernous haeman-
gioma (port-wine stain)

Other localized swellings in these regions include enlargement of the other salivary glands, lymphadenopathy and, particularly if inflamed and tender, abscesses.

Figure 19 Paget's disease causes excessive bone turnover and may lead to hypertrophy of the vault of the skull. It can also affect the spine and limbs (see **Figs 124, 191**).

Figure 20 Cavernous haemangioma is a hamartoma of mature capillary tissues. Distribution is variable but sometimes unilateral. Occasionally, it may be associated with a deeper lesion overlying the brain and this can be associated with developmental abnormalities and epileptic seizures (Sturge–Weber syndrome). Unlike the strawberry naevus, which regresses over the first few years of life, it is permanent.

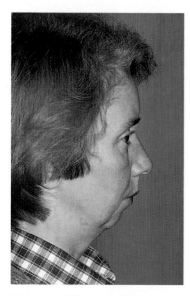

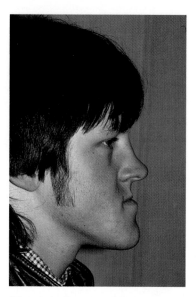

Fig. 21a Micrognathia   **Fig. 21b Prognathia**

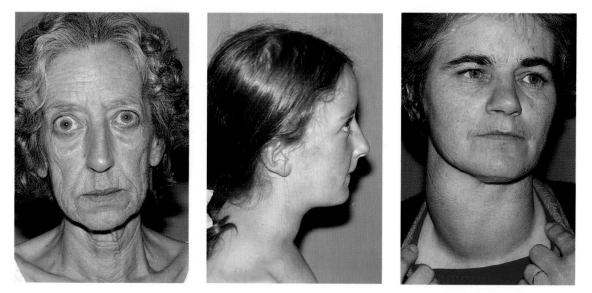

Fig. 22a Thyrotoxicosis   **Fig. 22b Goitre**   **Fig. 22c Goitre**

Figure 21a–b Abnormalities of the shape of the jaw can adversely affect chewing, speech and appearance. They may be constitutional or associated with disease that impairs normal growth. Micrognathia (**Fig. 21a**) describes a small mandible and prognathia (**Fig. 21b**) a protruding mandible. In both instances, there will be failure of the upper and lower teeth to meet effectively (dental malocclusion).

Figure 22a–c Thyroid disease may be associated with various features in the face and neck. A lean patient with eye signs (sclera visible all around the corneal limbus) demonstrates features of Graves' disease (**Fig. 22a**). Thyroid enlargement (goitre) may be subtle (**Fig. 22b**), or very obvious

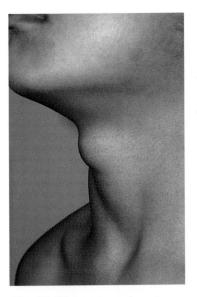

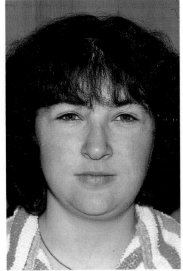

Fig. 23 Thyroglossal cyst   **Fig. 24a Hypothyroidism**

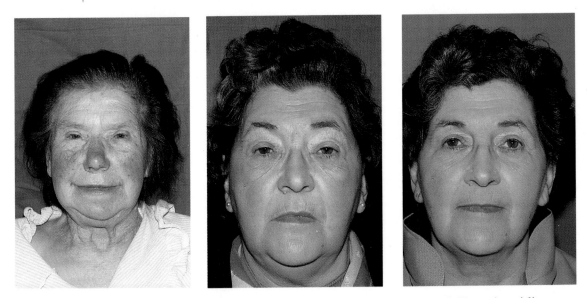

Fig. 24b Hypothyroidism   **Fig. 24c Hypothyroidism –**   **Fig. 24d Hypothyroidism –**
                                                  untreated   treated

(**Fig. 22c**) with swelling (not necessarily symmetrical) in the lower anterior neck which moves up and down on swallowing.

Figure 23 A thyroglossal cyst is a cystic swelling in the midline, usually above the larynx, which rises when the tongue is protruded.

Figure 24a–d Hypothyroidism produces thickening of soft tissues (**Fig. 24a**), thinning of the hair (**Fig. 24b**) and impairment of mental function. Institution of thyroxine therapy sometimes dramatically reverses the subtle facial features of this insidious condition (**Fig. 24c–d**).

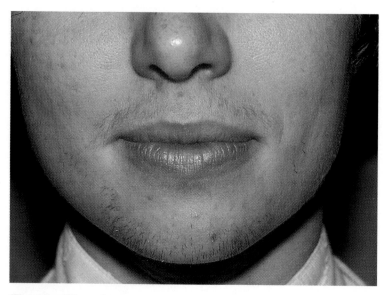

Fig. 25a Hirsutism

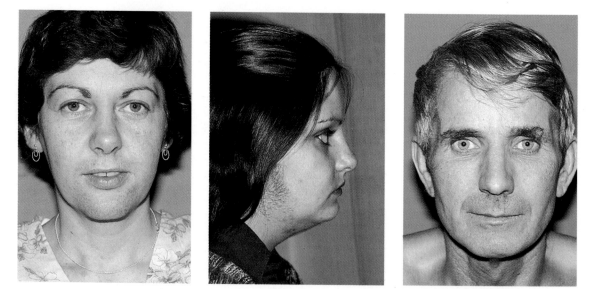

Fig. 25b Hirsutism   **Fig. 25c Hirsutism**   **Fig. 26 Addisonian pigmentation**

Figure 25a–c Hirsutism describes the presence of excessive facial hair in women. Its definition is somewhat subjective depending on racial and cultural norms. Distribution is typically on the upper lip and chin but can be more extensive. Evidence of shaving is sometimes more apparent than hirsutism and bleaching is often used for cosmetic effect.

Figure 26 Non-racial facial pigmentation may be seen in conditions associated with high adrenocorticotropic hormone (ACTH) levels (hypoadrenalism, Nelson's syndrome, ectopic ACTH syndrome), or may be drug induced (e.g. chlorpromazine).

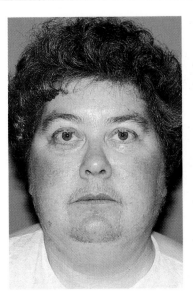

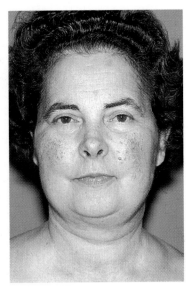

Fig. 27a Cushing's syndrome – spontaneous

Fig. 27b Cushing's syndrome – iatrogenous

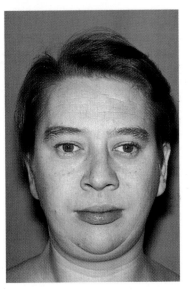

Fig. 28 Hypopituitarism (male)

Figure 27a–b Cushing's syndrome is due to excess circulating glucocorticoids. Increased deposition of fat in the cheeks and under the chin leads to the so-called (full) moon face (**Fig. 27a**) appearance and there may be associated telangiectasia (**Fig. 27b**). It is commonly drug induced in patients receiving glucocorticoid therapy. Pituitary-dependent Cushing's syndrome (also known as Cushing's disease) may also show the effects of adrenal androgen excess (hirsutism).

Figure 28 A hypopituitary male can exhibit features of androgen deficiency, e.g. smooth skin, increased subcutaneous fat, lack of facial hair and a female hairline (lack of temporal recession). This patient also exhibits an acquired divergent squint which has arisen due to suprasellar extension of a non-functioning pituitary tumour.

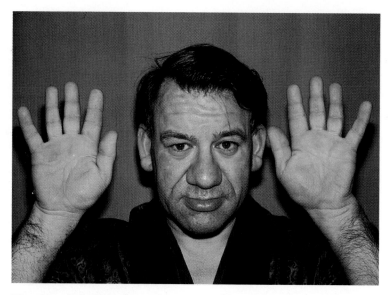

Fig. 29a Acromegaly

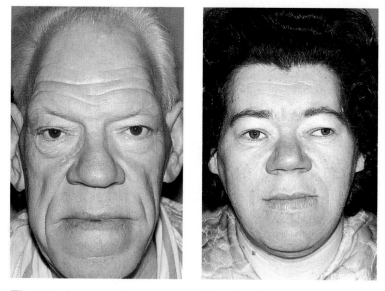

Fig. 29b Acromegaly   **Fig. 29c Acromegaly**

Figure 29a–c Acromegaly due to excess production of growth hormone by a pituitary tumour produces enlargement of the supraorbital ridges, thickening of lips and broadening of nose, prognathia and increased greasiness of the skin. **Figure 29a** also shows the broad, thick hands of acromegaly and **Figure 29c** the divergent squint of a partial third cranial nerve palsy associated with extrasellar pituitary tumour extenson.

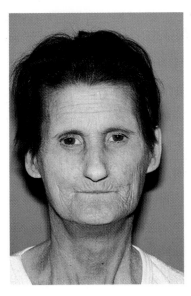

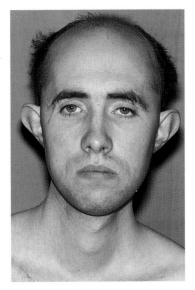

Fig. 30 Progressive systemic sclerosis

Fig. 31 Myotonic dystrophy

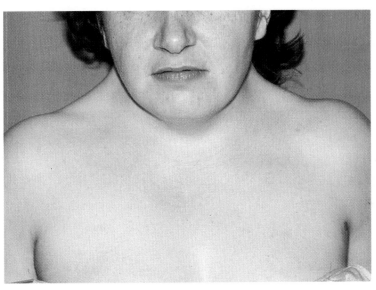

Fig. 32 Neck webbing

Figure 30 Progressive systemic sclerosis is a connective tissue disorder whose features include thickening and tightening of facial skin giving pinched features and perioral puckering. There is abnormal fixity of the skin.

Figure 31 Myotonic dystrophy is an autosomal dominant disorder of muscle and other tissues. Features include ptosis, horizontal mouth, wasted sternocleidomastoid and temporalis muscles and premature frontal balding.

Figure 32 Neck webbing, folds of skin and soft tissue running from the acromion to the side of the neck, is one feature of Turner's syndrome (45,XO). Other features include short stature, multiple melanotic naevi, cardiovascular abnormalities (including coarctation) and infertility.

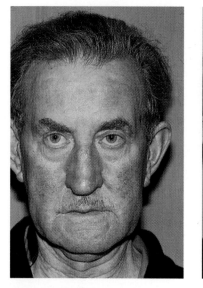

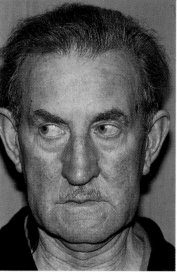

Fig. 33a Left sixth nerve
palsy – looking ahead

Fig. 33b Left sixth nerve
palsy – looking right

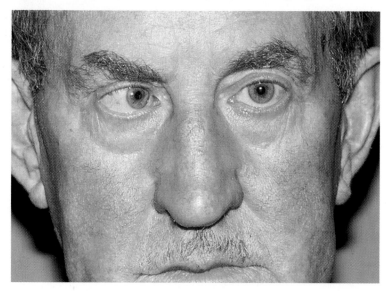

Fig. 33c Left sixth nerve palsy – looking left

Figure 33a–c Acquired or paralytic squint is normally the result of a mononeuropathy of many possible aetiologies. The patient complains of double vision only in some directions of gaze, the more peripheral image being produced by the 'weak' eye. In left sixth nerve palsy, forward (**Fig. 33a**) and right (**Fig. 33b**) gaze are normal but there is failure to abduct the left eye (due to left lateral rectus paralysis) on left gaze (**Fig. 33c**).

Fig. 34a Left third nerve palsy – looking right

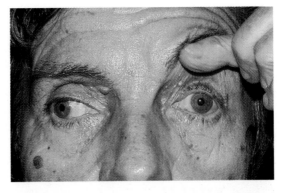

Fig. 34b Left third nerve palsy – complete ptosis

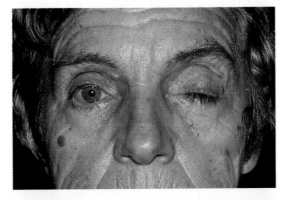

Fig. 34c Left third nerve palsy – pupillary dilatation

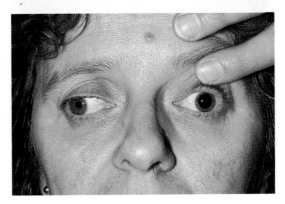

Figure 34a–c In third nerve palsy, the affected eye tends to look down and outward under the combined influence of the two extraocular muscles (lateral rectus and superior oblique) which are not supplied by the third nerve. In a complete third nerve palsy, there will also be ptosis (**Fig. 34b**) and pupillary dilatation (**Fig. 34c**).

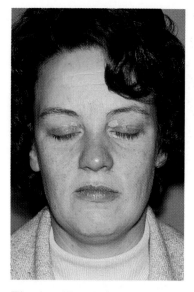

Fig. 35a Xanthelasmata

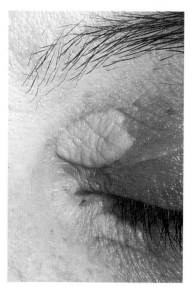

Fig. 35b Xanthelasmata

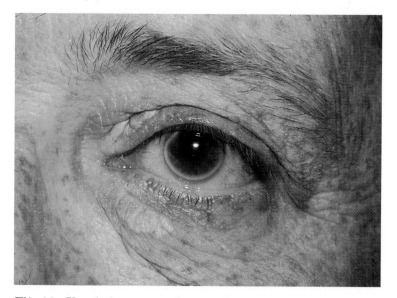

Fig. 35c Xanthelasmata and corneal arcus

Figure 35a–e Xanthelasmata are periorbital deposits of lipid-rich material. Their presence, particularly in younger individuals, should raise the suspicion of hyperlipidaemia. A corneal arcus in a young person may also indicate a lipid disorder.

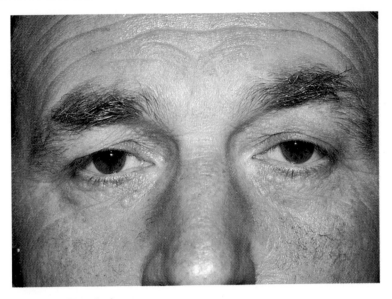

Fig. 35d Xanthelasmata

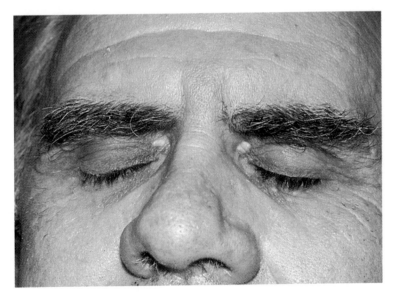

Fig. 35e Xanthelasmata

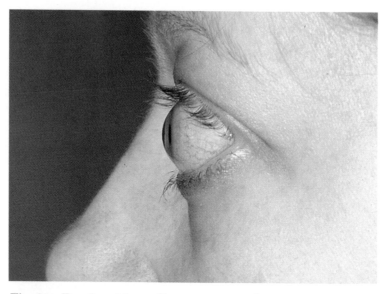

Fig. 36a Dysthyroid eye disease – proptosis

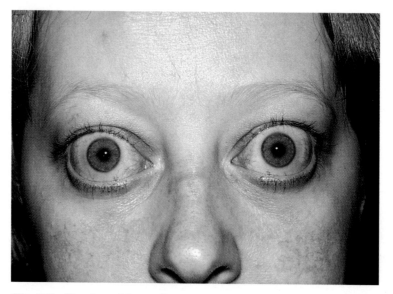

Fig. 36b Dysthyroid eye disease – upper and lower lid retraction

Figure 36a–b Dysthyroid eye disease is associated with swelling of the extraocular muscles. The resulting forward displacement of the eyeball (proptosis, **Fig. 36a**) leads to the appearance of sclera between the corneal limbus and the upper and lower eyelids (**Fig. 36b**). Inflammation of the conjunctiva may result. Exposure and subsequent dessication and ulceration of the cornea may ensue.

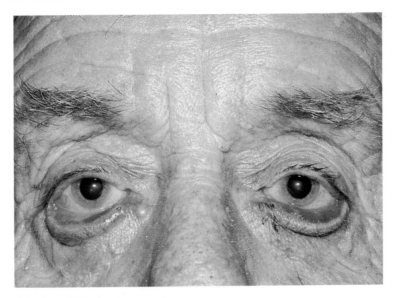

Fig. 37a Bilateral ectropion

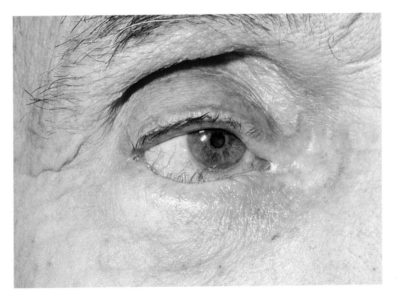

Fig. 37b Entropion

Figure 37a–b Increased skin laxity and loss of orbicularis oculi muscle tone due to age-related changes commonly leads to eyelid malposition. Eversion (ectropion, **Fig. 37a**) leads to impaired tear drainage (epiphora) while inversion (entropion, **Fig. 37b**) may result in corneal irritation and ulceration from inturned lashes.

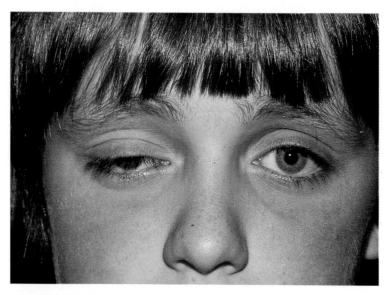

Fig. 38a Ptosis – congenital

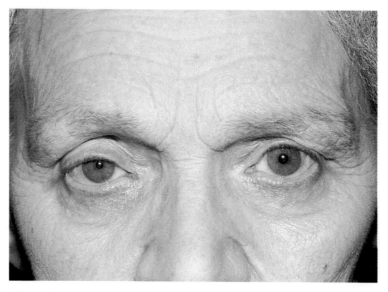

Fig. 38b Ptosis – acquired: Horner's syndrome

Figure 38a–b Ptosis is the term given to drooping of the eyelid. It may be congenital (**Fig. 38a**), in which case the lid fold in the skin is poorly developed, or acquired, e.g. due to third nerve palsy or damage to innervation. Impaired sympathetic innervation gives rise to Horner's syndrome (**Fig. 38b**) in which mild ptosis is accompanied by pupillary constriction and ipsilateral diminution of sweating.

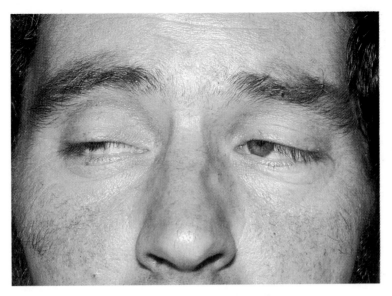

Fig. 39a Myasthenia gravis – bilateral ptosis

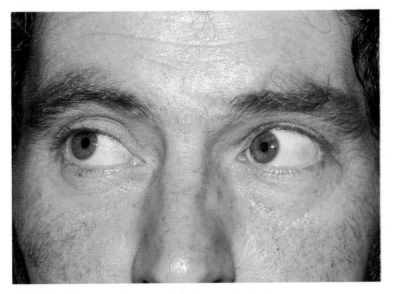

Fig. 39b Myasthenia gravis – after anticholinesterase injection

Figure 39a–b Intermittent ptosis, especially if bilateral (**Fig. 39a**), suggests the possibility of myasthenia gravis, in which case the ptosis should be rapidly (and temporarily) reversed (**Fig. 39b**) by intravenous injection of an anticholinesterase drug, such as edrophonium bromide.

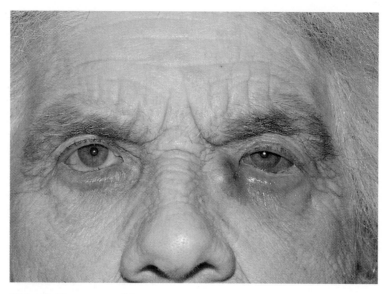

Fig. 40 Dacryocystitis

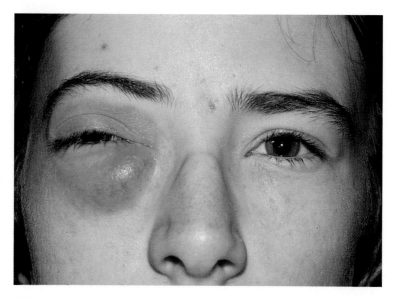

Fig. 41 Orbital cellulitis

Figure 40 Dacryocystitis is an infection of the lacrimal sac, which lies medial to the caruncle underneath the canthal tendon.

Figure 41 Orbital cellulitis is a more serious sight-threatening condition where signs of acute inflammation (erythema, swelling and tenderness) are present around the eye, and may extend backwards to compromise the optic nerve.

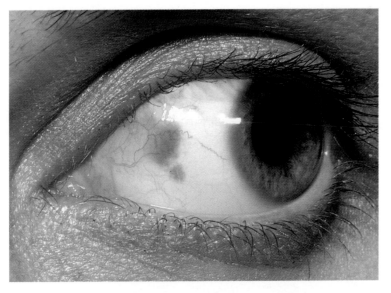

Fig. 42a Subconjunctival haemorrhage – spontaneous

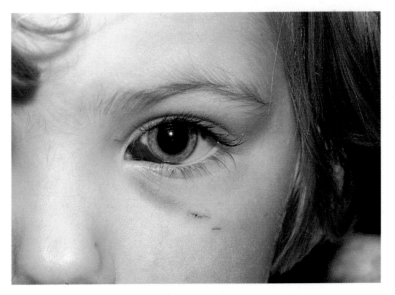

Fig. 42b Subconjunctival haemorrhage – traumatic

Figure 42a–b Subconjunctival haemorrhage has a dramatic appearance but is seldom serious. It consists of extravasation of blood beneath the conjunctiva, which takes several weeks to resolve. Such bleeding may be spontaneous (**Fig. 42a**) or traumatic (**Fig. 42b**) in its causation.

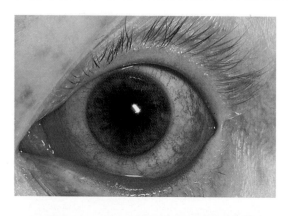

Fig. 43a Conjunctivitis –
limbal pallor

Fig. 43b Iritis – limbal
injection

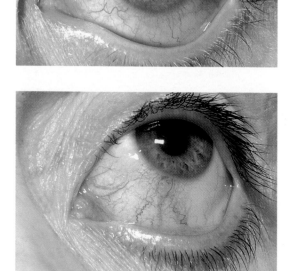

Fig. 44a Episcleritis

Figure 43a–b Conjunctivitis and iritis both produce 'red eyes'. The former is common and seldom serious – there is typically less redness around the corneal limbus (**Fig. 43a**). In contrast, the episcleral injection is more marked around the limbus in iritis (**Fig. 43b**).

Figure 44a–d Inflammation of the white coat of the eye (sclera and episclera) may be diffuse or nodular. Episcleritis (**Fig. 44a**) is a mild superficial inflammation, unlike scleritis (**Fig. 44b–c**) which is deeper, painful and sight threatening. The sclera may become thin (scleromalacia, **Fig. 44d**) and even perforate.

Fig. 44b Scleritis – nodular

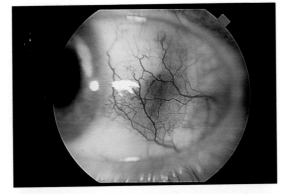

Fig. 44c Scleritis – diffuse

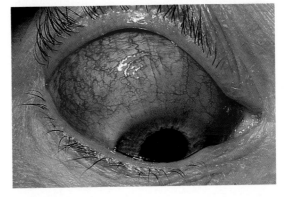

Fig. 44d Scleromalacia

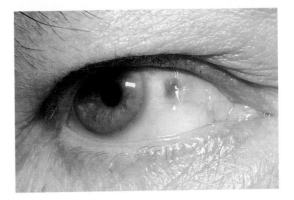

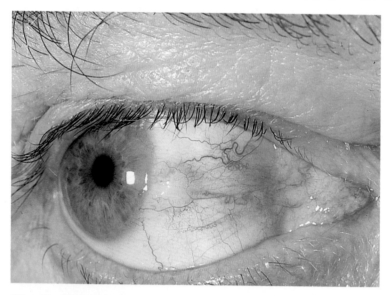

Fig. 45a Pinguecula

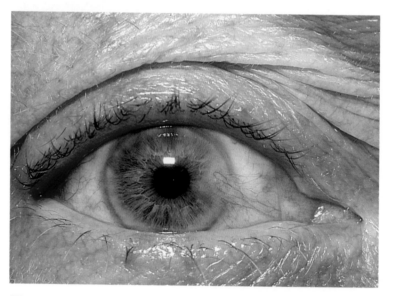

Fig. 45b Pterygium

Figure 45a–b A pinguecula (**Fig. 45a**) is a yellowish fatty-looking episcleral nodule of little clinical significance, which should be distinguished from a pterygium (**Fig. 45b**), which is a fibrovascular fold of tissue advancing slowly over the cornea.

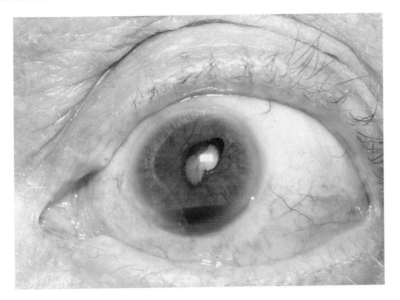

Fig. 46 Hyphaema

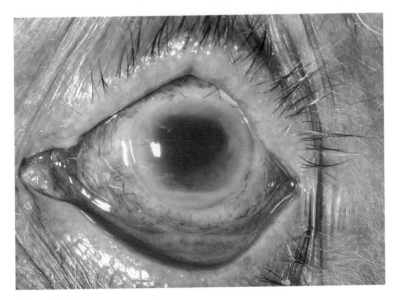

Fig. 47 Hypopyon

Figure 46 A hyphaema is blood in the anterior chamber of the eye, which may form a fluid level due to sedimentation. While a hyphaema may result from trauma, in this eye blood has leaked from new vessels on the iris (rubeosis iridis).

Figure 47 A hypopyon is pus in the anterior chamber, which sediments in the aqueous under the effects of gravity. In this eye, infection has followed cataract surgery.

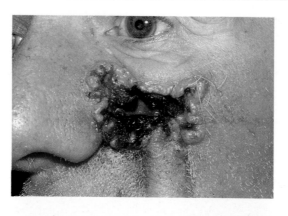

Fig. 48 Basal cell carcinoma (rodent ulcer)

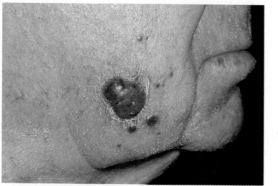

Fig. 49 Malignant melanoma

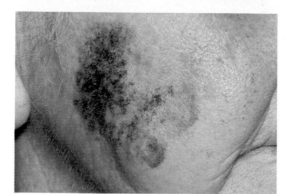

Fig. 50 Lentigo maligna

Figure 48 Basal cell carcinoma often occurs on the face. It begins as a firm nodule but can later spread with a rolled, pearly edge and central ulceration. This is an advanced example.

Figure 49 Malignant melanoma is characterized by a typically pigmented, enlarging or nodular lesion that may itch or bleed.

Figure 50 Lentigo maligna is a slowly-spreading pigmented naevus in sun-exposed areas in the elderly. These are premalignant lesions.

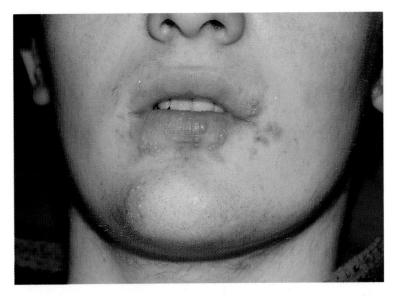

Fig. 51a Herpes simplex labialis

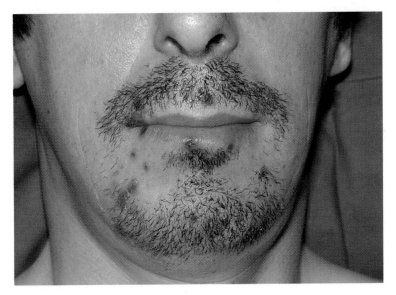

Fig. 51b Herpes simplex labialis

Figure 51a–b *Herpes Simplex Virus* infection is associated with tender vesicular lesions typically occurring in or around the lips (cold sores, **Fig. 51a**). They may occur during a systemic febrile illness, such as lobar pneumonia. Following rupture of the vesicles, scabs form (**Fig. 51b**).

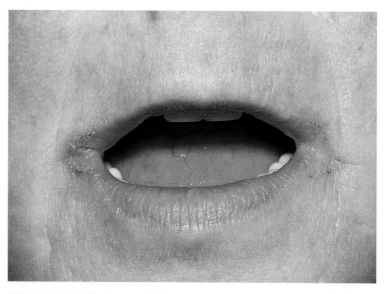

Fig. 52a Angular stomatitis

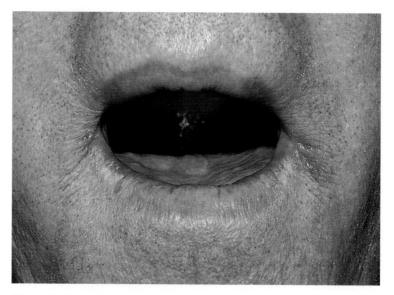

Fig. 52b Angular stomatitis

Figure 52a–b Angular stomatitis consists of red, sore, sometimes cracked skin at the corners of the mouth. It may be associated with nutritional deficiency, anaemia or ill-fitting dentures.

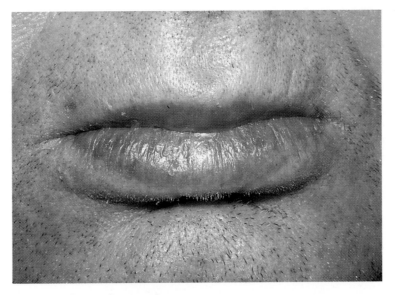

Fig. 53a Central cyanosis

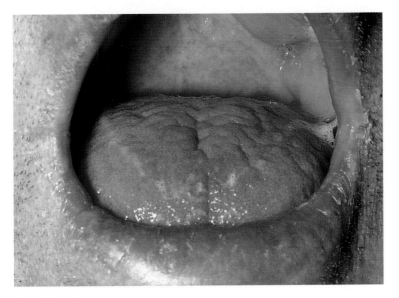

Fig. 53b Central cyanosis

Figure 53a–b Cyanosis is discoloration of tissues caused by high levels of desaturated haemoglobin. Central cyanosis seen in the lips or buccal mucosa indicates incomplete oxygenation of blood due to cardiac or respiratory disease, e.g. right to left cardiac shunt, chronic obstructive lung disease, fibrosing alveolitis and severe cases of asthma, pneumonia and tension pneumothorax. Peripheral cyanosis (see **Fig. 74**) may be present without central cyanosis, but not vice versa.

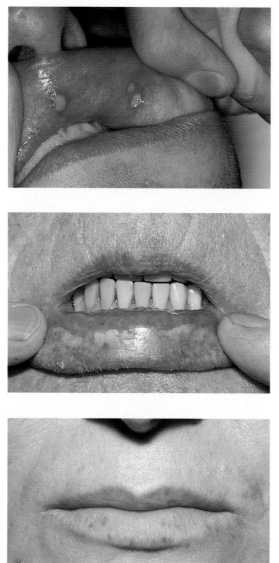

Fig. 54 Buccal ulceration

Fig. 55 Leukoplakia

Fig. 56 Pigmented spots: Peutz–Jeghers syndrome

Figure 54 Buccal ulceration, with painful, inflamed areas associated with defects in the normal buccal epithelium, is common and usually due to minor trauma. It can be a feature of several systemic diseases, e.g. connective tissue disorders and leukaemia, particularly when severe and protracted.

Figure 55 Leukoplakia consists of white, hyperkeratotic patches on the buccal mucosa with sharply demarcated edges. It often progresses to squamous carcinoma and is common in AIDS.

Figure 56 Pigmented freckles on and around the lips are characteristic of rare, hereditary gastrointestinal polyposis known as Peutz–Jeghers syndrome.

Fig. 57 Dental caries

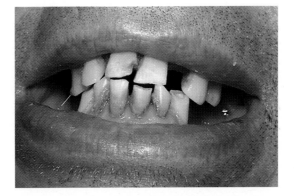

Fig. 58 Tetracycline staining

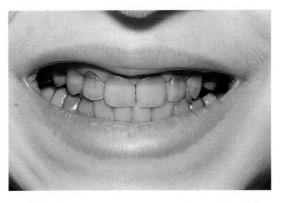

Fig. 59 Gum hyperplasia

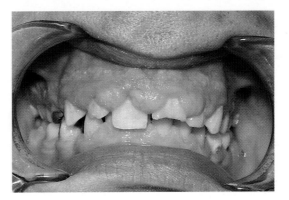

Figure 57 Dental caries is a bacterially mediated disease causing damage to mineral and organic components of teeth. The picture shows gum recession from periodontitis, loss of enamel, exposure of dentine and accumulation of discoloured tartar.

Figure 58 Tetracycline administered prior to maturation of the secondary dentition, i.e. before about 8 years of age, can lead to permanent discoloration and hypoplasia of dental enamel.

Figure 59 Overgrowth of the gums (gingival hyperplasia) is a feature of treatment with the anticonvulsant drug phenytoin. It is seldom functionally important.

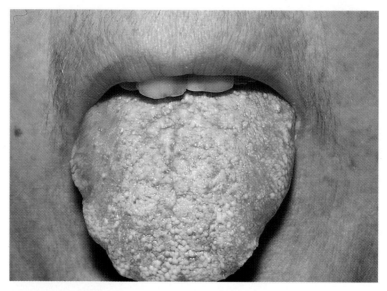

Fig. 60 Candidiasis

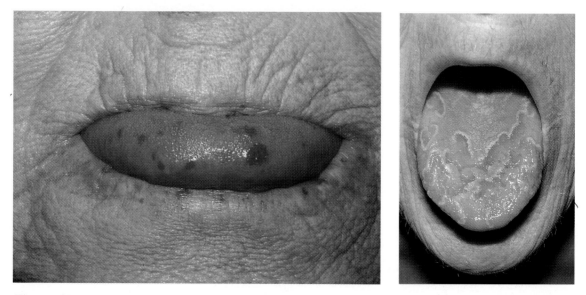

Fig. 61 Hereditary haemorrhagic telangiectasia   **Fig. 62 Geographic tongue**

Figure 60 *Candida* infection (thrush) can affect the tongue and palate (see **Fig. 67**) with mycelial plaques.

Figure 61 The multiple congenital telangiectatic lesions of hereditary haemorrhagic telangiectasia may be seen on the tongue, lips and fingers (see **Fig. 95**). If bleeding has been a major problem, there may be associated pallor.

Figure 62 Geographic tongue is usually asymptomatic and thus of little clinical significance once recognized. It is characterized by irregular patchy shedding of glossal papillae with sequential regrowth.

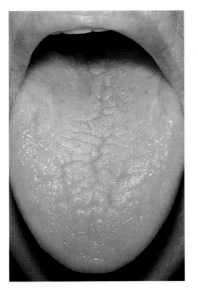

Fig. 63a Pallor

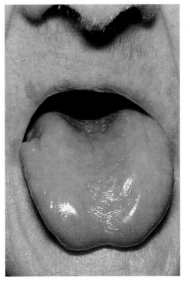

Fig. 63b Atrophic glossitis

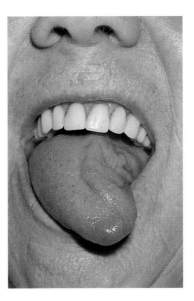

Fig. 64 Left twelfth-nerve palsy

Figure 63a–b Pallor of the tongue (**Fig. 63a**) is typical in anaemia of various causes. When due to vitamin B$_{12}$ or folate deficiency it is particularly likely to be accompanied by loss of the glossal papillae, giving a smooth (atrophic) appearance (**Fig. 63b**).

Figure 64 A lower motor neurone lesion of the left hypoglossal (twelfth) cranial nerve leads to ipsilateral wasting with fasciculation, and deviation of the tongue to the affected side on attempted protrusion.

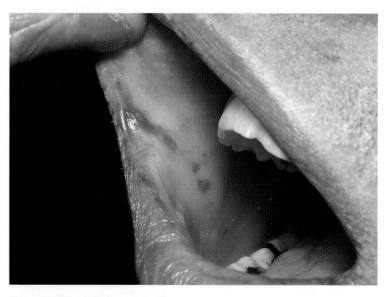

Fig. 65 Buccal pigmentation

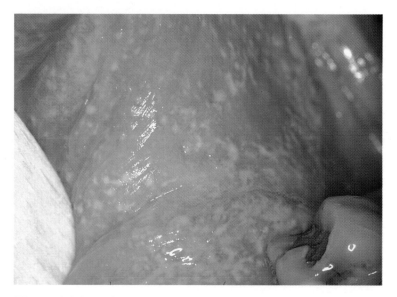

Fig. 66 Lichen planus

Figure 65 Melanotic pigmentation in the buccal mucosa, often along the line of dental closure, suggests an underlying diagnosis of primary hypoadrenalism (Addison's disease). There may be associated pigmentation of the face, hands and recent scars (see **Figs 26, 101** and **151** respectively).

Figure 66 Lichen planus can produce a characteristic buccal rash which may ulcerate.

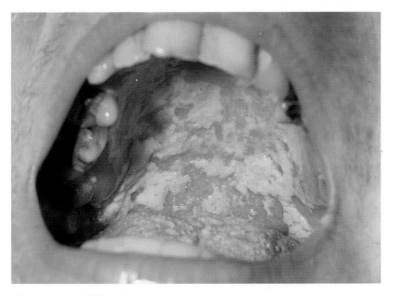

Fig. 67 Candidiasis

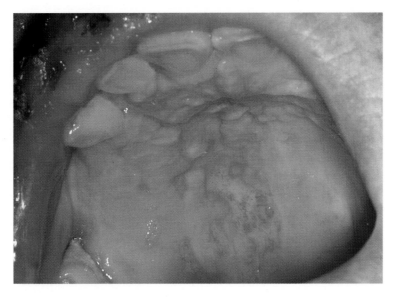

Fig. 68 Herpes zoster

Figure 67 Plaques of *Candida* infection may adhere to the palate and tongue (see **Fig. 60**).

Figure 68 *Herpes Zoster* affecting the maxillary division of the trigeminal nerve (see **Fig. 156**) will also produce painful vesicles and ulcers on the corresponding side of the palate.

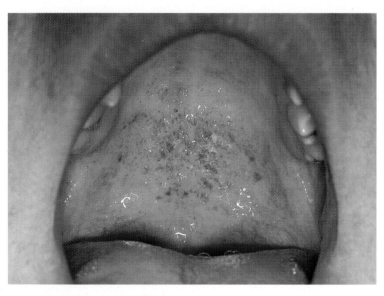

Fig. 69a Palatal petechiae

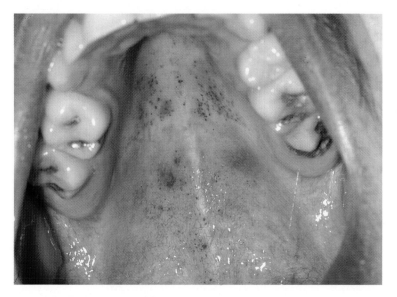

Fig. 69b Palatal petechiae

Figure 69a–b Palatal petechiae can be part of generalized petechiae, e.g. in association with thrombocytopenia, and can be a localized feature of viral infections, particularly infectious mono-nucleosis.

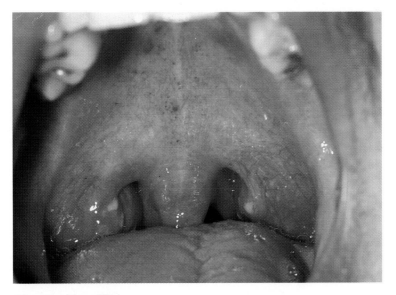

Fig. 70a Tonsillitis

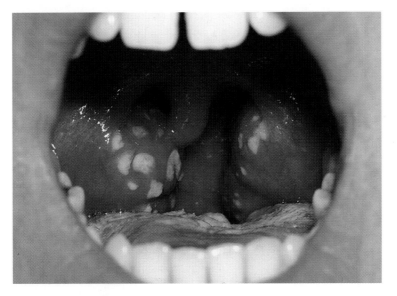

Fig. 70b Tonsillitis

Figure 70a–b Tonsillitis may be viral or, less commonly, bacterial (especially *Streptococcal*). The palate, uvula and tonsils show swelling and erythema and there may be white exudates or caseous material in pits on the tonsils. Palatal petechiae again suggest infectious mononucleosis.

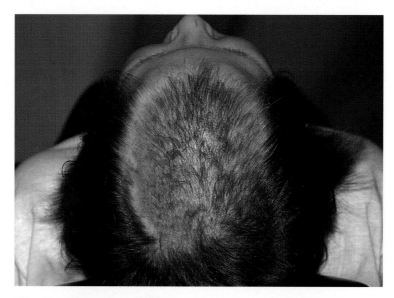

Fig. 71a Alopecia – diffuse

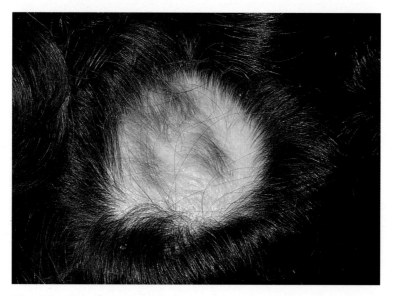

Fig. 71b Alopecia – patchy

Figure 71a–b Alopecia is hair loss which may be diffuse (**Fig. 71a**), causing thinning of the hair, or patchy (**Fig. 71b**) with scarring of the underlying scalp such as can occur in systemic lupus erythematosus and lichen planus.

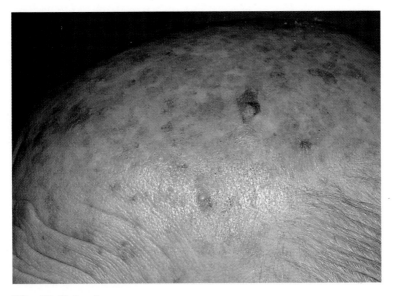

Fig. 72 **Solar keratoses**

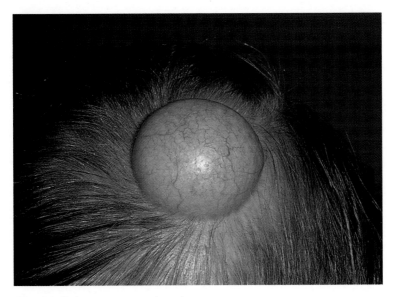

Fig. 73 **Sebaceous cyst (wen)**

Figure 72 Solar keratoses are lesions consisting of epidermal thickening leading to roughened areas of skin or sometimes inflammation. They occur in skin exposed to the sun and may progress to squamous carcinoma.

Figure 73 A sebaceous cyst of the scalp is sometimes referred to as a 'wen'. The swelling is fluctuant and painless and not inflamed, although there may be dilated vessels visible in the skin stretched over it.

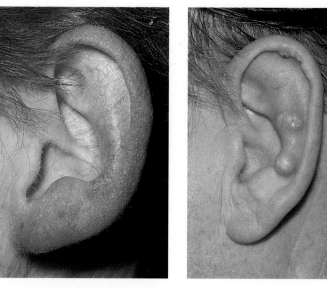

Fig. 74 **Peripheral cyanosis**   Fig. 75 **Gouty tophi**

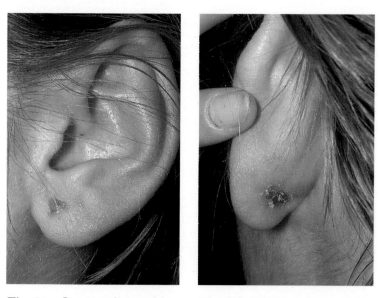

Fig. 76a **Contact dermatitis**   Fig. 76b **Contact dermatitis**

Figure 74 Cyanosis due to increased levels of circulating desaturated haemoglobin can be seen in several peripheral sites, including the pinnae. Warm extremities suggest the cyanosis is central, whereas primary peripheral cyanosis occurs when the extremities are cold.

Figure 75 Gouty tophi are painless, nodular collections of uric acid which may ulcerate. They can occur in many sites, including the ears.

Figure 76a–b Contact dermatitis to jewellery, especially nickel jewellery, can be responsible for the appearance of red, irritant, crusted lesions at either end of the track in a pierced ear lobe.

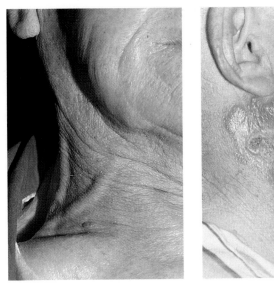

Fig. 77 **Distended neck veins**   Fig. 78 **Scrofula**

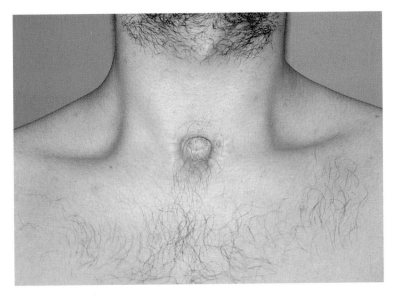

Fig. 79 **Tracheostomy scar**

Figure 77 Distended neck veins may indicate raised right heart pressure, e.g. cardiac failure or pericardial constriction. Superficial vessels, such as the external jugular veins illustrated here, may give an artificially high impression of central venous pressure if they are kinked or compressed on passing through deep fascia.

Figure 78 Scrofula is due to tuberculous cervical lymphadenopathy with chronic induration, ulceration and scaling.

Figure 79 A scarred, deep pit in the jugular notch is a typical sequel to tracheostomy.

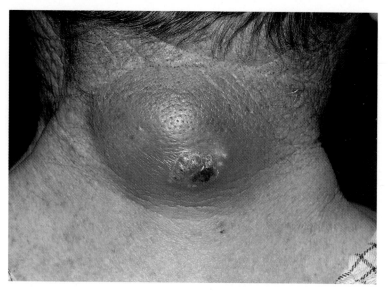

Fig. 80 Carbuncle

Figure 80 Carbuncles can occur at any site but most often where minor peripheral trauma can allow entry of microorganisms. Typically due to *Staphylococcus aureus* infection, the lesion shows all the features of acute inflammation (erythema, swelling, warmth, tenderness) and typically points with leakage of pus if the overlying skin breaks or is incised.

2 Hands, arms and axillae

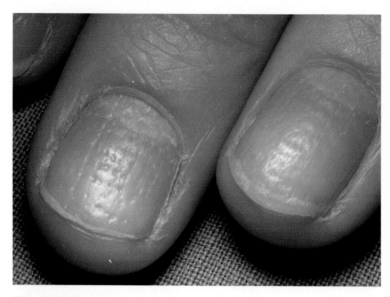

Fig. 81 Nail pitting

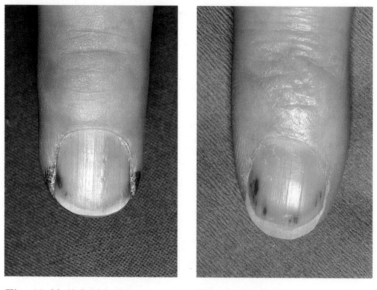

Fig. 82 Nail fold infarcts   **Fig. 83 Splinter haemorrhages**

Figure 81 Nail pitting – a series of small dimples on the surface of the nail – is a feature of psoriasis (see **Fig. 219**) and occurs less commonly in association with dermatitis and alopecia areata.

Figure 82 Nail fold infarcts may indicate an underlying vasculitic process as can occur in some connective tissue diseases, e.g. seropositive rheumatoid disease.

Figure 83 Splinter haemorrhages are linear red, brown or black marks usually occurring near the free edge of the nail. They are most commonly isolated and result from minor trauma. Greater numbers are a clue to underlying microembolic disease, especially bacterial endocarditis.

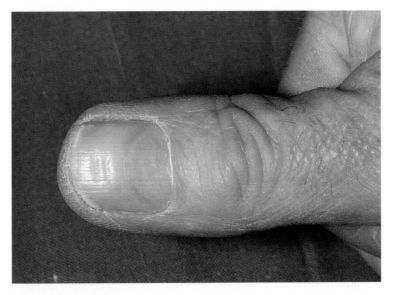

Fig. 84 Beau's lines

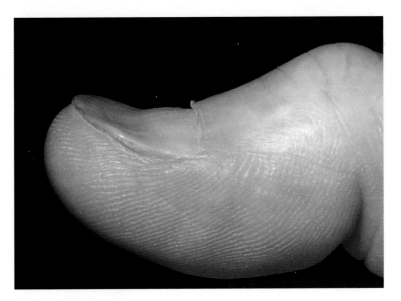

Fig. 85 Koilonychia

Figure 84 Beau's lines are transverse depressions on the nail consistent with a non-specific episode of illness. Their appearance can retrospectively indicate such an occurrence.

Figure 85 Koilonychia, or spooning of the nails, occurs when the normal upward convexity becomes a concavity. Rarely congenital, koilonychia is a feature of chronic iron deficiency.

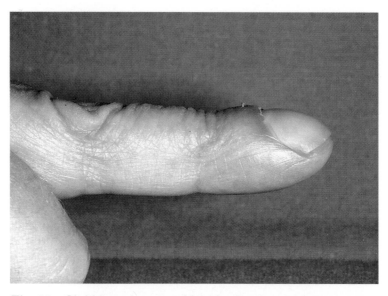

Fig. 86a Clubbing – increased longitudinal curvature

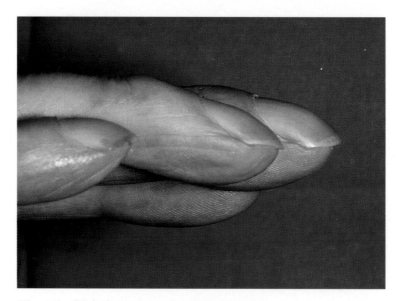

Fig. 86b Clubbing – loss of nail-bed angle

Figure 86a–c Clubbing consists of increased longitudinal (**Fig. 86a**) and transverse nail curvature, loss of the normal angle between the nail and nail bed (**Fig. 86b**) and increased fluctuation of the nail on the underlying soft tissues. At its most severe, clubbing is associated with a bulbous thickening of the terminal phalangeal soft tissue producing a drumstick-like appearance (**Fig. 86c**). While it can be congenital and innocent, clubbing has many disease associations including bronchial carcinoma, chronic pulmonary suppuration, fibrosing alveolitis, infective endocarditis, congenital cyanotic heart disease, inflammatory bowel disease and thyrotoxicosis.

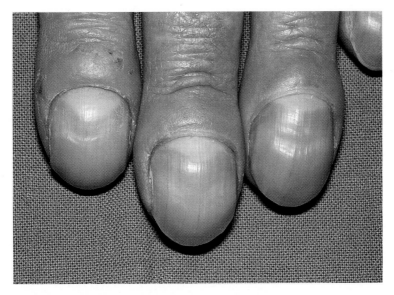

Fig. 86c Clubbing – drumstick appearance

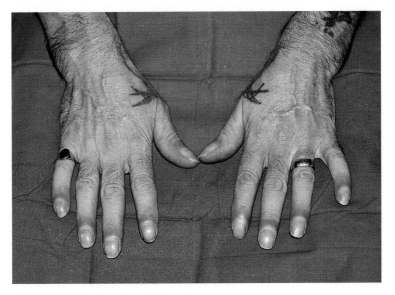

Fig. 87 Periungual erythema

Figure 87 Periungual erythema, or redness around the nail beds, is a feature of some connective tissue diseases, e.g. scleroderma. Dilated capillaries may be apparent on close inspection.

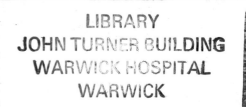

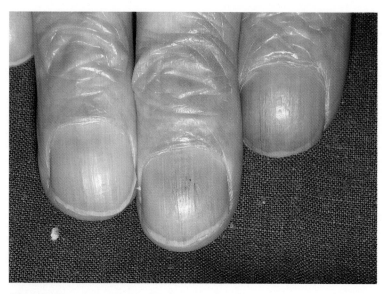

Fig. 88 Tar (nicotine) staining

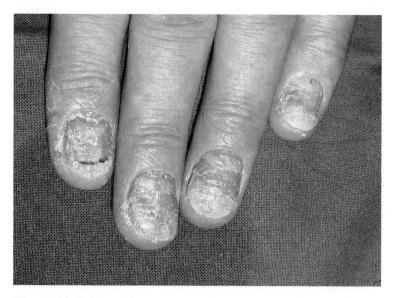

Fig. 89 Nail dystrophy

Figure 88 Tar stains from tobacco are often found on the finger nails of habitual smokers. (Nicotine is colourless and hence the popular reference to 'nicotine staining' is erroneous.)

Figure 89 Nail dystrophy, or abnormal structure and form of the nail, occurs in various conditions, including psoriasis (see **Fig. 219**) and fungal infection.

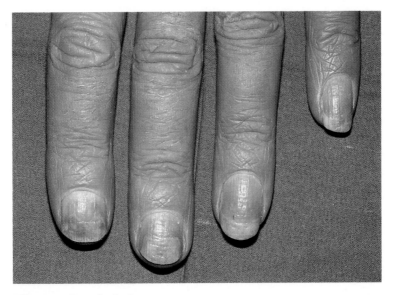

Fig. 90a Onycholysis

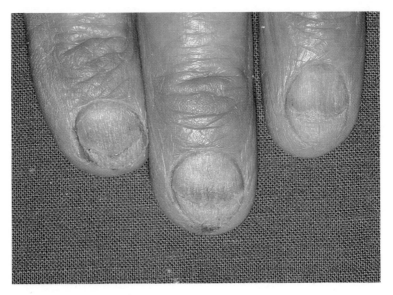

Fig. 90b Onycholysis

Figure 90a–b Separation of the nail from the nail bed, or onycholysis, usually begins distally and may occur in psoriasis, fungal infection, thyrotoxicosis and following trauma.

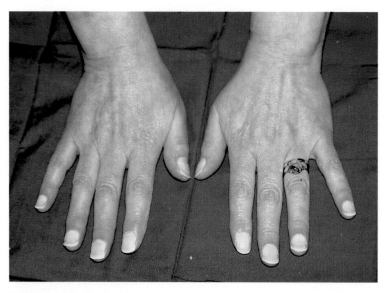

Fig. 91a Leukonychia

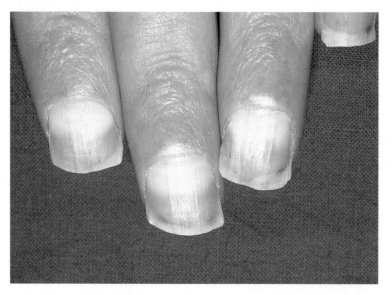

Fig. 91b Leukonychia

Figure 91a–b Leukonychia, or white nails, are seen in hypoalbuminaemic disorders, such as malnutrition, malabsorption, hepatic disease and nephrotic syndrome. When the hypoproteinaemia is intermittent, the nails may show partial or variable whitening, the white areas having developed while low albumin levels prevailed.

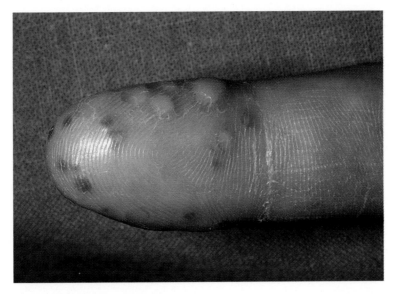

Fig. 92 Herpetic whitlows

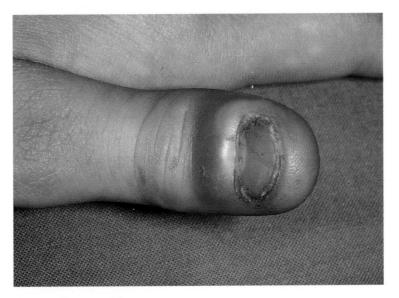

Fig. 93 Paronychia

Figure 92 Herpetic whitlow is the term given to a vesicle/pustule in the finger tip due to *Herpes Simplex* infection. It is acutely tender. These lesions are differentiated from simple furuncles by their tendency to vesiculate and occur in crops.

Figure 93 Acute paronychia is an infection, usually *Staphylococcal*, around the edge of the nail with redness and extreme tenderness. Pus may be visible under the skin of the nail fold and beneath the nail plate itself.

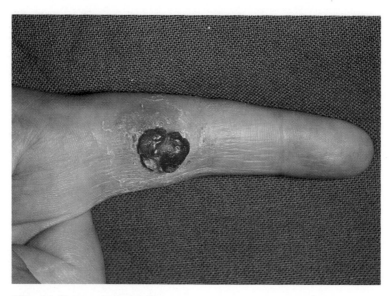

Fig. 94 Pyogenic granuloma

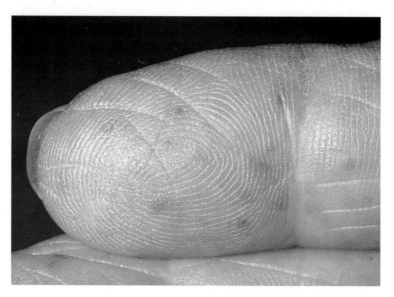

Fig. 95 Hereditary haemorrhagic telangiectasia

Figure 94 A pyogenic granuloma is an irregular, nodular, vascular lesion which is typically painless and which develops at the site of trauma. It is prone to bleeding on minimal trauma.

Figure 95 Hereditary haemorrhagic telangiectasia is characterized by multiple submucosal or subcutaneous lesions that may be apparent in the fingers or mouth (see **Fig. 61**).

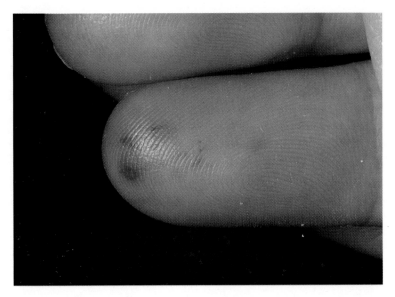

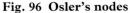

Fig. 96 Osler's nodes

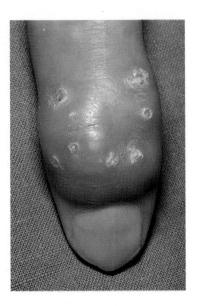

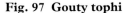

Fig. 97 Gouty tophi

Figure 96 Osler's nodes are tender, normally indurated, lesions in the finger pulp, classically associated with infective endocarditis and possibly due to embolization of debris from the diseased valve. A similar phenomenon occurring on the palm is referred to as a Janeway lesion.

Figure 97 Tophi are subcutaneous deposits of uric acid seen in chronic hyperuricaemia. They occur in various sites including the ears (see **Fig. 75**), and may ulcerate and discharge their contents.

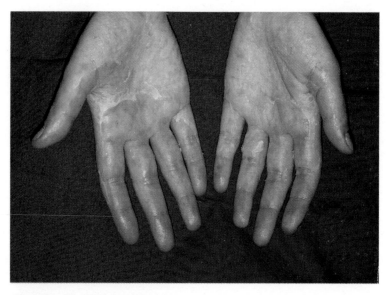

Fig. 98a Desquamation

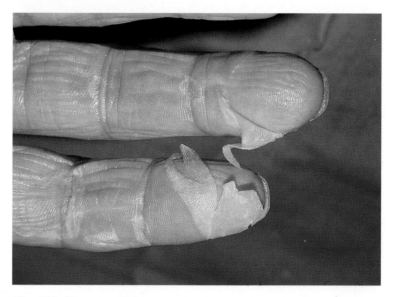

Fig. 98b Desquamation

Figure 98a–b Desquamation, or peeling of the skin, is common as a local occurrence around a focal lesion. It can also be more generalized after infective episodes, especially *Streptococcal* infection.

Fig. 99 Psoriatic arthropathy and nail dystrophy

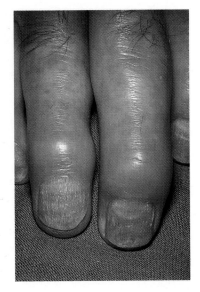

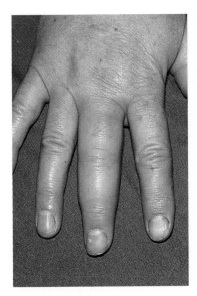

Fig. 100a Dactylitis – psoriatic

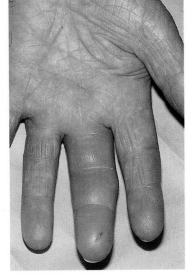

Fig. 100b Dactylitis – infective

Figure 99 Psoriasis (see **Fig. 215**) may cause nail dystrophy and pitting, and may be associated with digital arthritis, especially involving the distal interphalangeal joints.

Figure 100a–b Dactylitis, or inflammation of a digit, is normally a feature of psoriatic arthropathy (**Fig. 100a**). Soft-tissue infection, often with a penetrating wound, can give rise to an infective dactylitis (**Fig. 100b**).

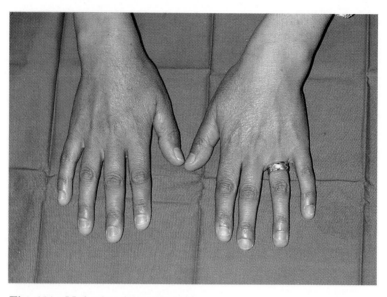

Fig. 101a Melanin pigmentation

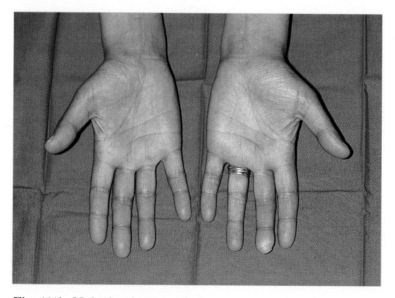

Fig. 101b Melanin pigmentation

Figure 101a–b Melanin pigmentation may be due to racial origin, but when marked over the knuckles and in the palmar creases in fair-skinned individuals, it may be an indication of elevated ACTH levels. Look also for ACTH-related pigmentation on the buccal mucosa (see **Fig. 65**), in immature scars (see **Fig. 151**) and at sites of chronic pressure, e.g. bra straps and waist belts.

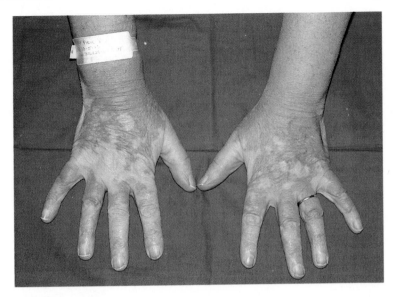

Fig. 102 Vitiligo

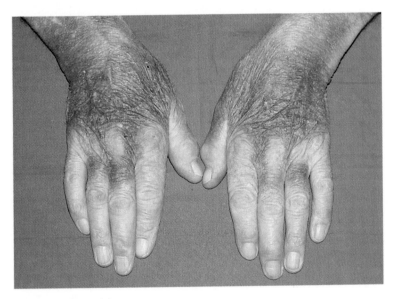

Fig. 103 Steroid purpura

Figure 102 Vitiligo is a patchy or confluent loss of melanin pigmentation that is most often apparent in the hands. It is accentuated when sun exposure leads to tanning of normal skin, thus increasing the contrast.

Figure 103 Exposure to supraphysiological (usually exogenously administered) levels of glucocorticoids can lead to skin atrophy with an associated weakness of dermal capillaries resulting in recurrent or chronic purpura. Repeated dermal bleeding leads to accumulation of brownish haemosiderin in local tissues.

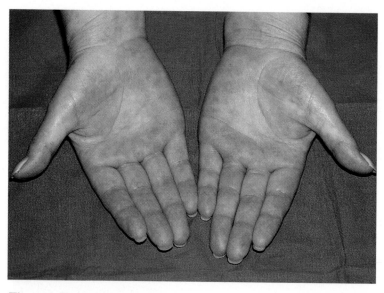

Fig. 104 **Palmar erythema**

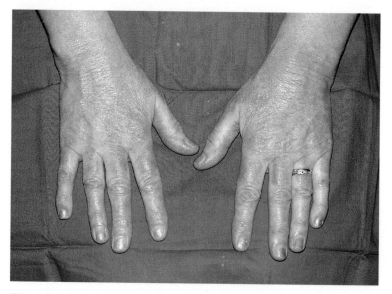

Fig. 105 **Dermatomyositis**

Figure 104 Palmar erythema shows as a blotchy redness of the palm, sparing the central area. It is associated with various conditions, including hepatic disease, hence its alternative name of 'liver palms'.

Figure 105 Dermatomyositis is a connective tissue disease involving both skin and muscle. It produces so-called 'heliotrope' discoloration of the periorbital skin and on the dorsum of the hands and fingers.

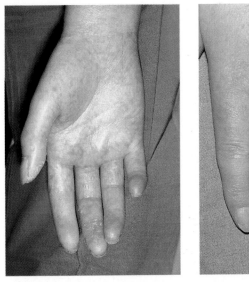

Fig. 106a Scleroderma

Fig. 106b Scleroderma

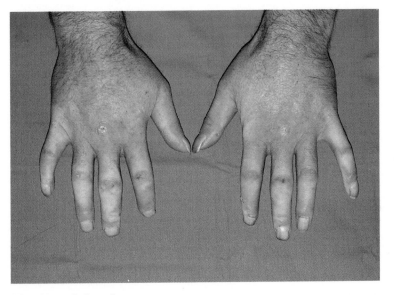

Fig. 106c Scleroderma

Figure 106a–c Scleroderma is a connective tissue disease that can have several manifestations in the hands, including oedema, thickened and taut skin, telangiectasia (especially around the nail folds), vasculitic infarcts and terminal digital gangrene with tissue resorption or amputation. **Figure 106c** shows calcinosis over some of the knuckles. There may also be characteristic facial features (see **Fig. 30**).

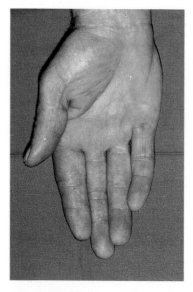

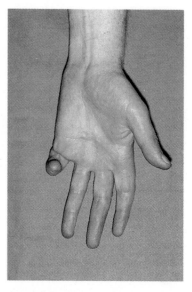

Fig. 107a Dupuytren's contracture

Fig. 107b Dupuytren's contracture

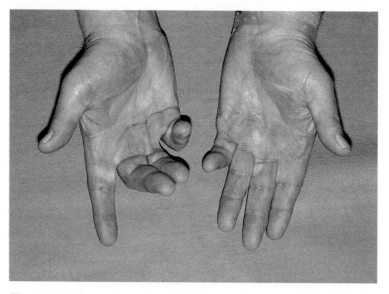

Fig. 107c Dupuytren's contracture

Figure 107a–c Dupuytren's contracture is characterized by thickened fibrous contracture of the palmar fascia. In its mild or early form, this may consist of palpable thickening and perhaps some puckering (normally overlying the fourth and fifth metacarpal). It can progress to produce a fixed flexion deformity of the fingers and is often bilateral, although asymmetrical. It is sometimes associated with alcoholic liver disease.

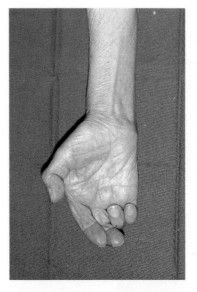 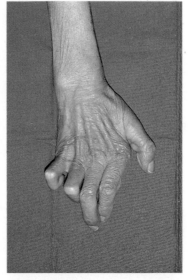

**Fig. 108a Ulnar nerve palsy
– claw hand**

**Fig. 108b Ulnar nerve palsy
– claw hand**

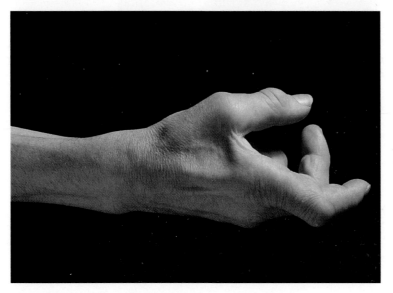

Fig. 109 Muscle wasting – first dorsal interosseus

Figure 108a–b Ulnar nerve palsy causes weakness and wasting of hand muscles resulting in ulnar claw hand deformity with hypothenar wasting, hyperextension of the fourth and fifth metacarpophalangeal joints and flexion of the related digits.

Figure 109 Muscle wasting of the hands is often first visible when the normal muscle bulk of the first dorsal interosseous muscle is replaced by a hollow.

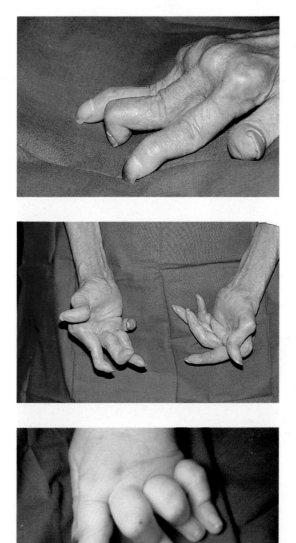

Fig. 110a Rheumatoid arthritis – swan-neck deformities

Fig. 110b Rheumatoid arthritis – swan-neck and Z-thumb deformities

Fig. 110c Rheumatoid arthritis – boutonnière deformities

Figure 110a–e Rheumatoid disease can produce multiple and varied abnormalities in the hands. The swan-neck deformity (**Fig. 110a–b**) is a descriptive term for the damage to tendon insertions that results in hyperextension of the proximal, and flexion of the distal, interphalangeal joints. In the boutonnière (buttonhole) deformity (**Fig. 110c**), destruction of the central attachment of the long extensor tendon to the middle phalanx leads to a flexion deformity of the proximal interphalangeal joint, the latter peeping through the 'buttonhole' bounded by the parts of the long tendon passing either side of the joint en route for the terminal phalanx. A similar lesion at the first metacarpophalangeal joint produces the self-explanatory Z-thumb deformity (**Fig. 110b**).

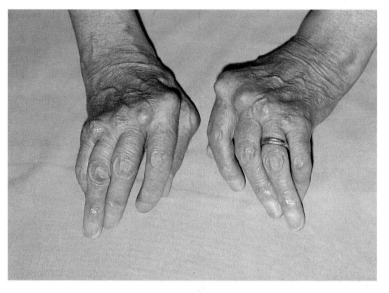

Fig. 110d Rheumatoid arthritis – ulnar deviation

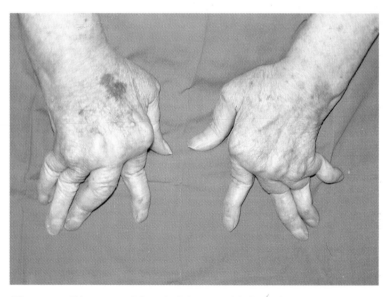

Fig. 110e Rheumatoid arthritis – multiple deformities

Subluxation of the metacarpophalangeal joints leads to prominence of the metacarpal heads with apparent joint swelling and ulnar deviation of the fingers (**Fig. 110d**). Sometimes many of these abnormalities, and digital osseous resorption with 'telescoping' of the digit, are combined (**Fig. 110e**). Steroid purpura and skin atrophy may also be present if it has been necessary to use this form of therapy. The distal interphalangeal joint is typically uninvolved in the disease.

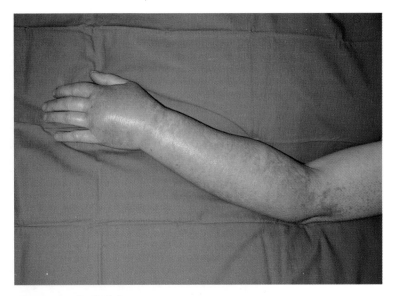

Fig. 115a Cellulitis

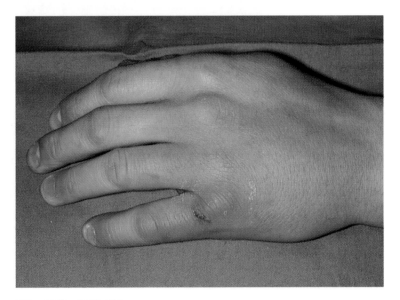

Fig. 115b Cellulitis

Figure 115a–b Cellulitis, or soft-tissue infection, produces erythema, tenderness and tense swelling. A puncture site where the offending organism (usually *Streptococcal*) gained entry may be obvious (**Fig. 115b**).

Fig. 116 Track marks ('mainlining')

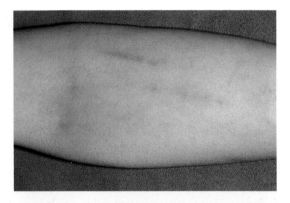

Fig. 117a Lymphangitis

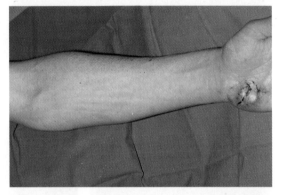

Fig. 117b Lymphangitis

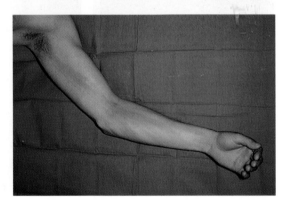

Figure 116 Repeated needling and superficial inflammation of veins, such as occurs with intravenous drug abuse, typically shows 'track marks' of haemosiderosis along the veins that have been involved.

Figure 117a–b Spread of infection (usually *Streptococcal*) from a wound may produce streaks of erythema due to inflammation of draining lymphatics.

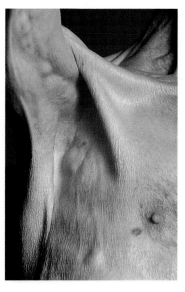

Fig. 126a Lymphadenopathy

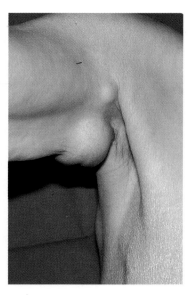

Fig. 126b Lymphadenopathy

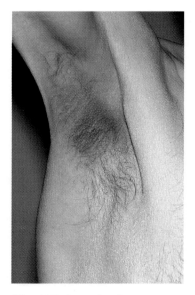

Fig. 127 Acanthosis
nigricans

Fig. 128 Pseudoacanthosis
nigricans

Figure 126a–b Enlargement of lymph nodes, or lymphadenopathy, may be apparent at sites of lymph node aggregation, such as the axilla. Unless the nodes are markedly enlarged, this will only be visible when subcutaneous fat is sparse.

Figure 127 In acanthosis nigricans, the skin is thickened and pigmented with melanin. This can be associated with intra-abdominal malignancy.

Figure 128 Pseudoacanthosis nigricans is simple pigmentation of flexural skin, usually in obese individuals. It is not associated with internal disease.

3 Chest, abdomen and genitalia

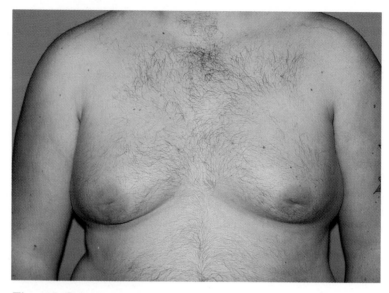

Fig. 129 Gynaecomastia

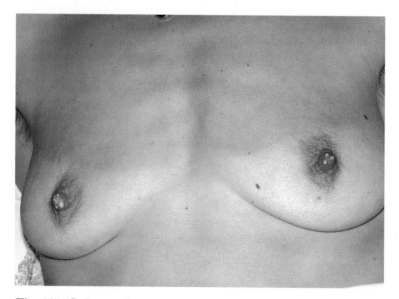

Fig. 130 Galactorrhoea

Figure 129 Gynaecomastia is mammary gland swelling in the male. It has many causes, including hepatic cirrhosis and puberty as well as drug therapy, e.g. spironolactone, cimetidine, digoxin and oestrogen.

Figure 130 Galactorrhoea is the inappropriate production and let down of breast milk, i.e. in a woman who is not currently breast feeding.

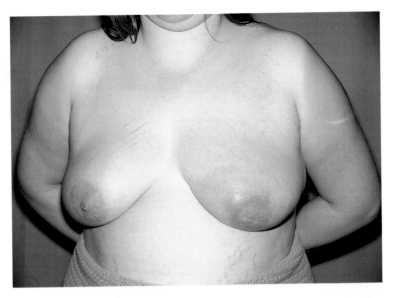

Fig. 131 Breast abscess

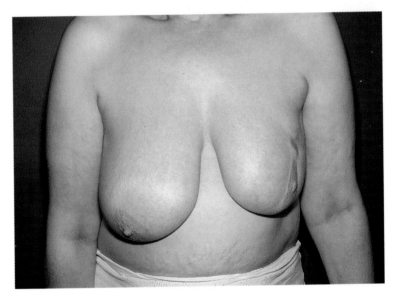

Fig. 132 Breast carcinoma

Figure 131 Firm, red, tender breast lesions, especially in suckling mothers, suggest breast abscess.

Figure 132 Breast carcinoma is often associated with contraction of fibrotic tissue around the lesion, which can produce breast asymmetry.

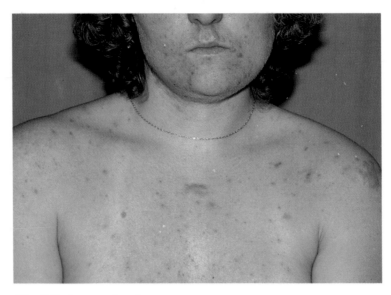

Fig. 147 Acne vulgaris

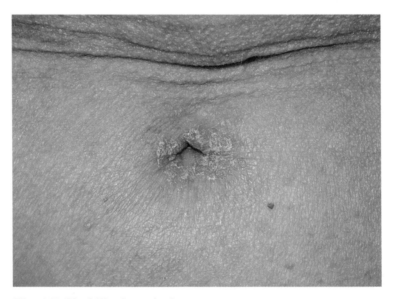

Fig. 148 Umbilical psoriasis

Figure 147 Acne vulgaris, characterized by facial comedones and inflamed skin spots with pustule formation, can sometimes spread on to the upper trunk.

Figure 148 Patients with psoriasis sometimes develop this typical scaling lesion in the periumbilical skin.

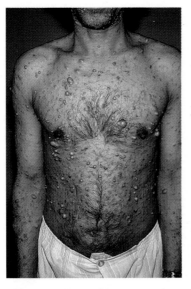

Fig. 149 Neurofibromatosis

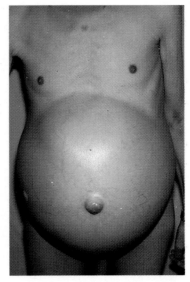

Fig. 150 Abdominal distension with everted umbilicus

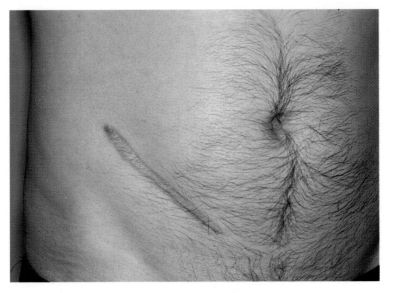

Fig. 151 Pigmented scar: Addison's disease

Figure 149 In florid examples of neurofibromatosis, multiple subcutaneous neurofibromata are present.

Figure 150 Abdominal distension with umbilical eversion can be a feature of cirrhosis or several types of intra-abdominal neoplasia. Distended veins radiating (and draining) away from the umbilicus – the so-called 'caput medusae' – indicate portal hypertension.

Figure 151 Melanin pigmentation developing in a scar, particularly if immature, suggests primary hypoadrenalism (Addison's disease).

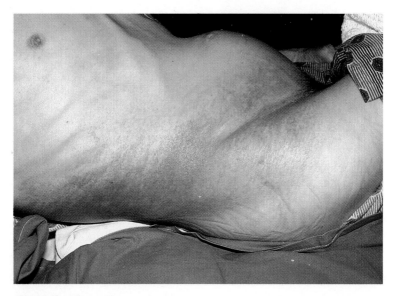

Fig. 152a Grey Turner's sign

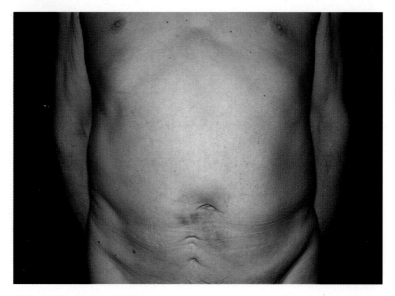

Fig. 152b Cullen's sign

Figure 152a–b Acute haemorrhagic pancreatitis can lead to tracking of extravasated blood into the flanks (Grey Turner's sign, **Fig. 152a**) or to the periumbilical region (Cullen's sign, **Fig. 152b**). These may also be seen following retroperitoneal bleeding from other causes, e.g. leaking aortic aneurysm.

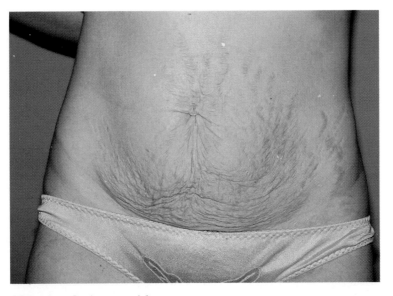

Fig. 153a Striae gravidarum

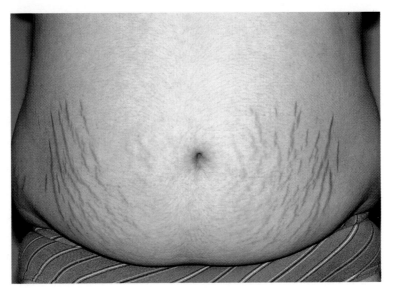

Fig. 153b Striae: Cushing's syndrome

Figure 153a–b Disruption of dermal collagen can lead to the development of abnormal streaks or striae that are roughly concentric upon the umbilicus. After the stretching by a gravid uterus, these are white and scarred (**Fig. 153a**), but in situations of glucocorticoid excess, e.g. Cushing's disease, the unduly fragile collagen is disrupted showing purplish-pink striae (**Fig. 153b**).

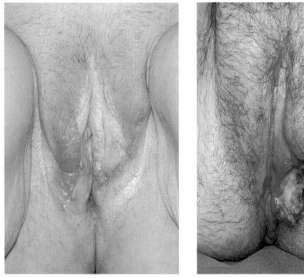

Fig. 168 Lichen sclerosus   Fig. 169 Vulval ulcer

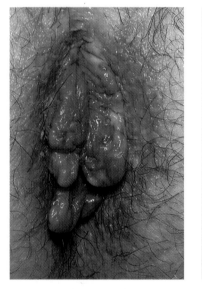

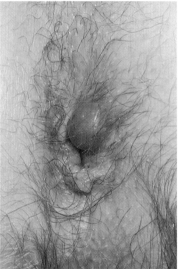

Fig. 170a Prolapsed   Fig. 170b Thrombosed
haemorrhoids   haemorrhoid

Figure 168 Lichen sclerosus consists of white, wrinkled skin patches often occurring in the vulvar region and sometimes complicated by squamous carcinoma.

Figure 169 Vulval ulceration has a number of causes, including *Herpes Simplex Virus* infection and carcinoma. It may also occur in association with aphthous ulceration in the mouth as part of Behçet's disease.

Figure 170a–b Varicosities of the internal haemorrhoidal veins can prolapse beneath the anal margin (**Fig. 170a**). Occasionally, acutely tender thrombosis will develop in one varix (**Fig. 170b**).

4 Legs and feet

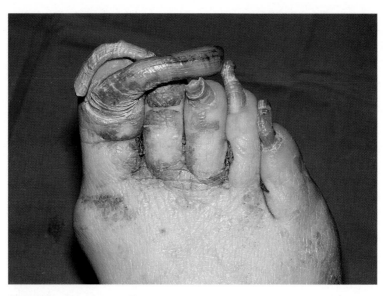

Fig. 171 Onychogryphosis

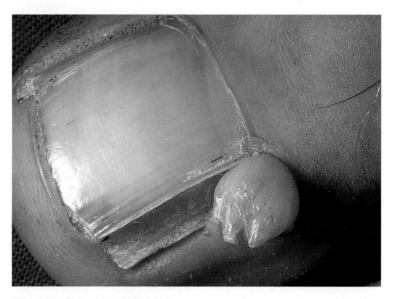

Fig. 172 Subungual fibroma

Figure 171 Onychogryphosis is thickening of the nail, most often seen with claw-like overgrowth in cases of prolonged neglect in the elderly. Hypertrophy may also occur following repeated trauma.

Figure 172 Subungual fibromata may develop around puberty in patients with the inherited disorder, tuberous sclerosis or epiloia. The typical facial lesions are shown in **Figure 14**.

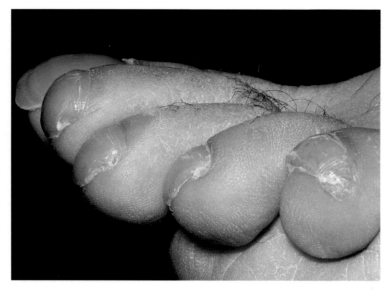

Fig. 173 **Clubbing**

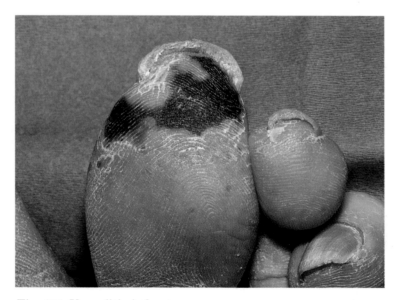

Fig. 174 **Vasculitic infarcts**

Figure 173 Clubbing of the toes has similar features and causes to finger clubbing with which it often coexists and which is described on page 52 (see **Fig. 86a–b**).

Figure 174 Vasculitis can lead to peripheral small-vessel occlusion resulting in dark, tender, often irregular areas of infarction. Lesions are likely to be multiple.

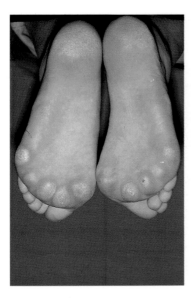

Fig. 178 Rheumatoid arthritis – metatarsophalangeal subluxations

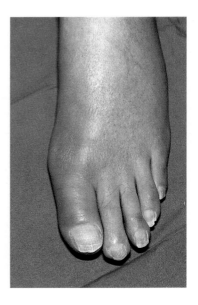

Fig. 179 Acute gout

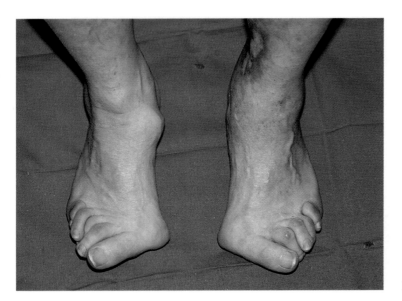

Fig. 180 Hallux valgus

Figure 178 Rheumatoid disease with subluxation of the metatarsophalangeal joints leads to callus formation under the metatarsal heads.

Figure 179 In acute gout, deposition of uric acid crystals within a joint (commonly the first metatarsophalangeal joint), leads to erythema, swelling (note shiny skin) and extreme pain on any attempt at movement of the joint. The diagnosis can be established by demonstrating uric acid crystals on joint aspiration.

Figure 180 Hallux valgus refers to deformity at the first metatarsophalangeal joint causing the great toe to deviate laterally. Exostoses commonly occurring at the medial side of the joint in this situation are popularly known as bunions.

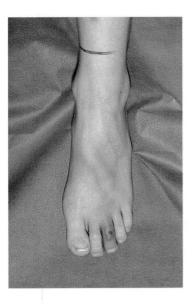

Fig. 181 Lymphangitis

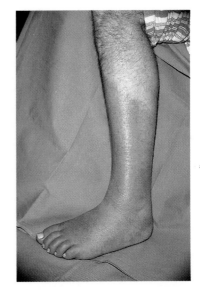

Fig. 182a Cellulitis

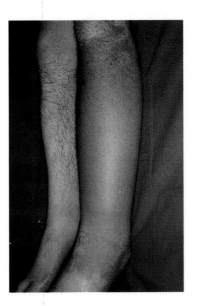

Fig. 182b Cellulitis –
acute

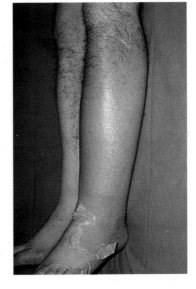

Fig. 182c Cellulitis –
resolving

Figure 181 Lymphangitis shows as red streaks of inflammation extending proximally from an infected wound. There may be associated inguinal lymph node enlargement and tenderness.

Figure 182a–c Cellulitis, or soft-tissue infection, most commonly occurs in the legs (**Fig. 182a**). The likeliest causal organism is a beta haemolytic *Streptococcus*. The site of entry is not always apparent; careful inspection of nail folds for evidence of an ingrowing toe nail may help in this situation. In the acute phase, the leg is bright red, swollen and tender (**Fig. 182b**). With resolution, the redness becomes duller, the swelling subsides leading to wrinkling of the skin, and extensive desquamation sometimes occurs over the affected area (**Fig. 182c**). Subcutaneous crepitus may indicate the less common, but potentially more serious, infection with a gas-forming organism (e.g. *Clostridium* species).

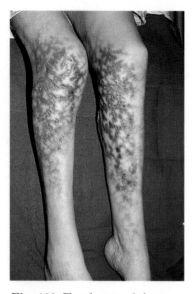

Fig. 183 Erythema ab igne

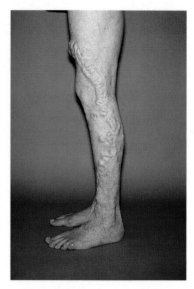

Fig. 184 Varicose veins

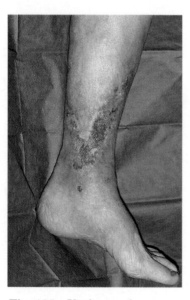

Fig. 185a Varicose ulcer

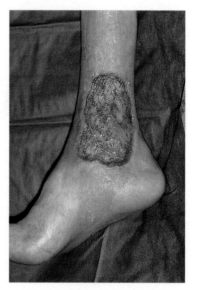

Fig. 185b Varicose ulcer

Figure 183 Erythema ab igne (literally redness from the fire) is a brownish, reticular skin rash occurring in response to chronic heat exposure, typically in an old person who sits close to the fire. In the case illustrated, the patient clearly sat with the fire habitually on her right side.

Figure 184 Varicose veins have incompetent valves leading to tortuous subcutaneous swellings. These are normally warm due to their blood content and there may be associated haemosiderin pigmentation as a result of chronic leakage of the red cells into the adjacent skin.

Figure 185a–b Varicose eczema and skin ulceration are complications of varicose veins and typically occur above the medial malleolus.

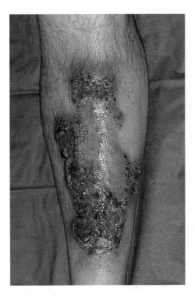

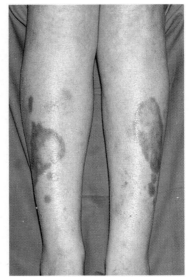

Fig. 186 Vasculitic ulceration

Fig. 187 Necrobiosis lipoidica

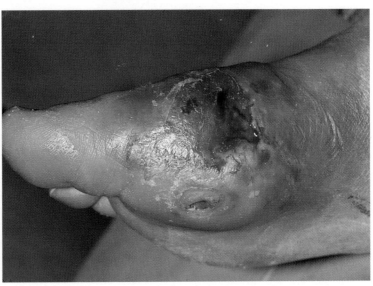

Fig. 188 Trophic ulceration

Figure 186 Vasculitic ulceration is associated with dark areas of vasculitic infarction. In the legs, it is most likely to become extensive over the tibia where the blood supply to the skin is normally at its most vulnerable.

Figure 187 Necrobiosis lipoidica consists of well-demarcated, yellow-brown plaques, often with depressed centres, which most commonly occur on the shins of young women with diabetes. The lesions are asymptomatic but may be cosmetically significant.

Figure 188 Trophic ulceration is often due to failure to protect the relatively anaesthetic neuropathic foot, e.g. in diabetic neuropathy, from the repeated stresses of walking. It typically affects areas of major pressure, e.g. under the ball of the foot and on the medial aspect of the first metatarsophalangeal joint, where tight-fitting shoes are worn.

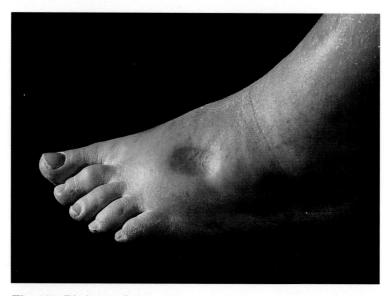

Fig. 189 Pitting oedema

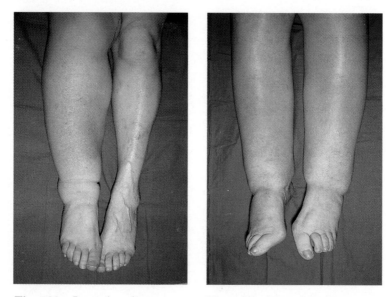

Fig. 190a Lymphoedema   Fig. 190b Lymphoedema

Figure 189 Accumulation of subcutaneous fluid (oedema) will leave a pit when pressed with the thumb for a few seconds. It occurs in various situations including venous insufficiency, hypo-albuminaemia and right-sided cardiac failure. Hypoalbuminaemic oedema characteristically refills quickly, i.e. within 30–60 seconds.

Figure 190a–b Lymphoedema is non-pitting and due to lymphatic obstruction. It may be unilateral. There are many causes, including lymphatic obstruction by malignancy or parasites, and the condition is often idiopathic in which case marked swelling of the foot is unusual.

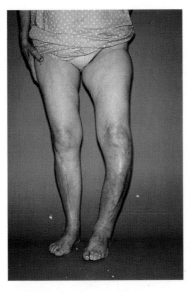

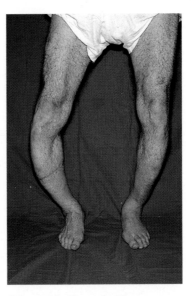

Fig. 191a Paget's disease

Fig. 191b Paget's disease

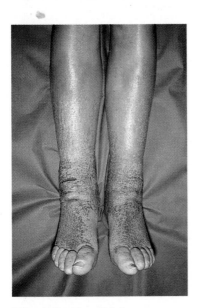

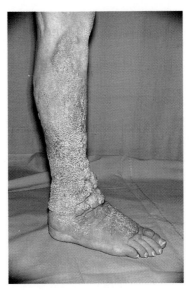

Fig. 192a Pretibial myxoedema

Fig. 192b Pretibial myxoedema

Figure 191a–b Paget's disease is associated with hypermetabolism of bone and can result in considerable bony deformity. Note that in both cases shown this deformity is confined to the bones in the lower leg and is not the typical bowing of rickets, which would also affect the femur.

Figure 192a–b Pretibial myxoedema produces a plaque-like, non-pitting swelling of the skin usually on the front of the legs and ankles, sometimes extending on to the dorsum of the foot. The skin is stretched over the underlying tissue, which may have an irregular, almost polypoid pattern (**Fig. 192b**). The condition occurs in association with Graves' disease.

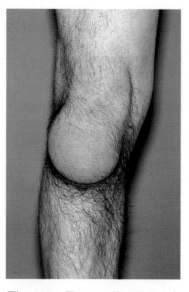

Fig. 193a Prepatellar bursa

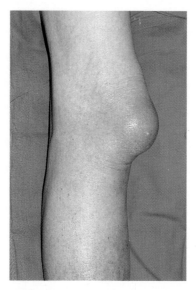

Fig. 193b Prepatellar bursitis

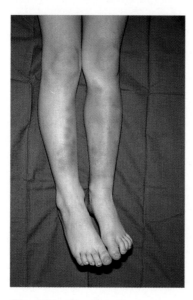

Fig. 194a Erythema nodosum

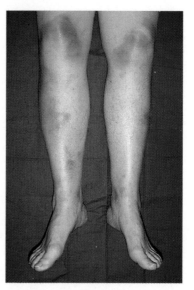

Fig. 194b Erythema nodosum

Figure 193a–b The large prepatellar bursa (**Fig. 193a**) is prone to trauma, especially on repeated kneeling, and can become swollen and tender (housemaid's knee). Inflammation or infection (usually following a puncture wound) is referred to as bursitis (**Fig. 193b**).

Figure 194a–b Erythema nodosum produces reddish, indurated, tender lesions of varying extent and most commonly on the shins. The rash is associated with many conditions including *Streptococcal* or primary *Tuberculous* infection, sarcoidosis, inflammatory bowel disease, sulphonamides and oestrogen.

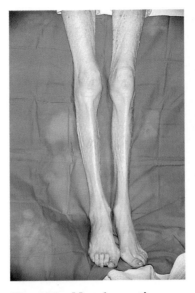

Fig. 195a Muscle wasting –
cachexia

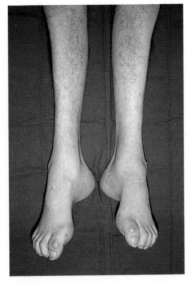

Fig. 195b Muscle wasting –
neuropathic

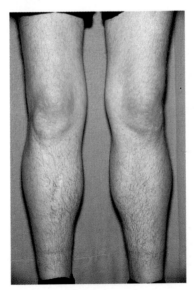

Fig. 196a Muscular dystrophy
– pseudohypertrophy

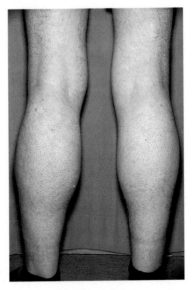

Fig. 196b Muscular dystrophy
– pseudohypertrophy

Figure 195a–b Severe muscle wasting (**Fig. 195a**) may be a feature of malignant disease or malnutrition, including anorexia nervosa or malabsorption. Symmetrical distal muscle wasting with preservation of proximal muscles is likely to be due to a hereditary or acquired peripheral neuropathy (**Fig. 195b**).

Figure 196a–b In some types of muscular dystrophy, apparent muscle hypertrophy (pseudo-hypertrophy) is none the less associated with weakness. There is probably true hypertrophy of some fibres while there is atrophy of others and fat infiltration. This appearance in the legs is typical of Becker muscular dystrophy in adults and Duchenne muscular dystrophy in children.

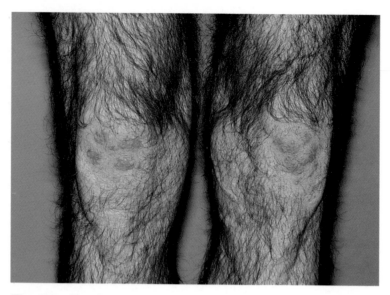

Fig. 197a Xanthomata

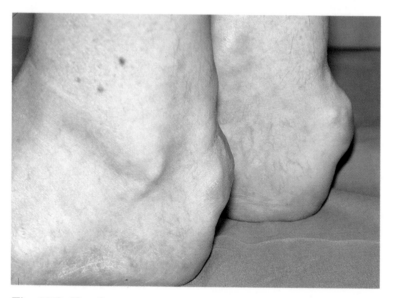

Fig. 197b Xanthomata

Figure 197a–b Deposits of cholesterol-rich material in hyperlipidaemia can give rise to papular eruptive xanthomata in the skin (**Fig. 197a**) or larger deposits in tendons (**Fig. 197b**). Xanthomata appearing on the hands and arms can be seen in **Figure 125a–c**.

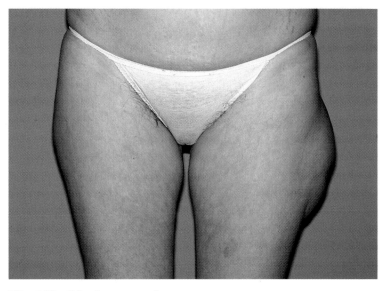

Fig. 198a Lipohypertrophy

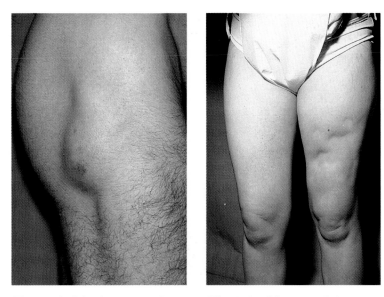

Fig. 198b Lipohypertrophy   Fig. 198c Lipoatrophy

Figure 198a–c Localized fat dystrophy – hypertrophy or atrophy – is associated with insulin therapy and leads to abnormal skin contours. Lipohypertrophy (**Fig. 198a–b**) commonly occurs when the patient repeatedly injects into the same localized area of skin. Lipoatrophy (**Fig. 198c**), thought to be due to an immunological reaction to injected insulin components, has become less common with the advent of more highly-purified insulin preparations.

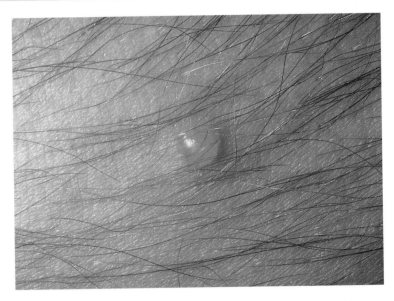

Fig. 204a Vesicle

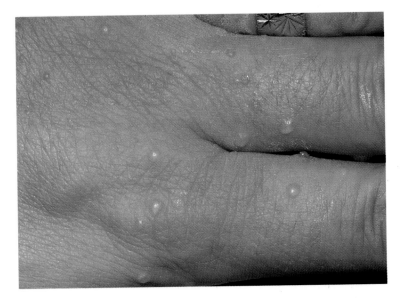

Fig. 204b Vesicles

Figure 204a–b A vesicle is a small, fluid-filled lesion on the skin in which serous fluid has separated the epidermis and dermis. Multiple lesions of this type can produce a vesicular eruption in certain viral infections.

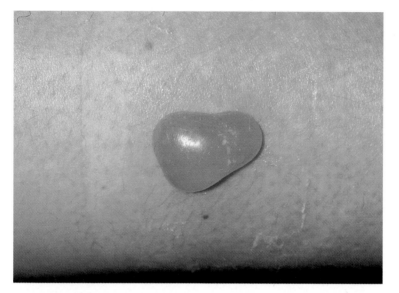

Fig. 205a Bulla

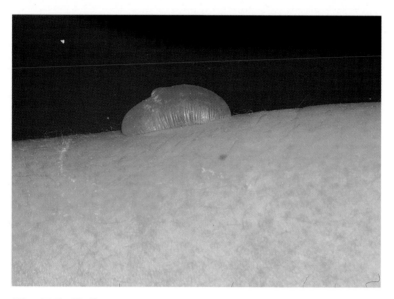

Fig. 205b Bulla

Figure 205a–b A bulla is a larger lesion that may contain considerable quantities of serous fluid. The fluid may be beneath the epidermis alone as in pemphigus (superficial) or collect intradermally as in pemphigoid (deep). Bullous eruptions can also occur with eczema, drug allergy, insect bites, etc.

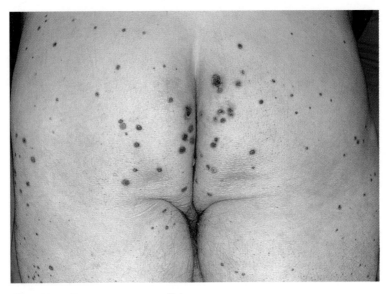

Fig. 206a Purpura – vasculitic

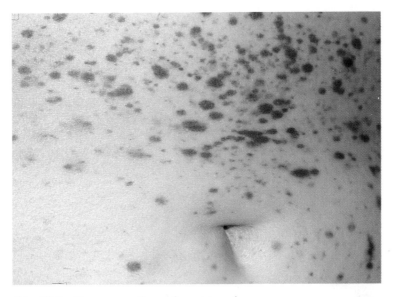

Fig. 206b Purpura – thrombocytopenic

Figure 206a–c Vasculitic purpura (**Fig. 206a**) is characterized by small intradermal extravasations of blood associated with small-vessel inflammation. The associated induration makes vasculitic purpura typically palpable. Henoch–Schönlein purpura is a relatively common form of this condition. Thrombocytopenic purpura (**Fig. 206b**) occurs in association with severe depression of platelet count and may be aggravated by minor trauma or locally raised tissue pressure. The lesions are impalpable. Senile purpura (**Fig. 206c**) is associated with fragility of capillaries and supporting connective tissues in the skin of the elderly. It typically produces blotchy lesions on the back of the hands and forearms.

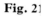

Fig. 21

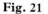

Fig. 21

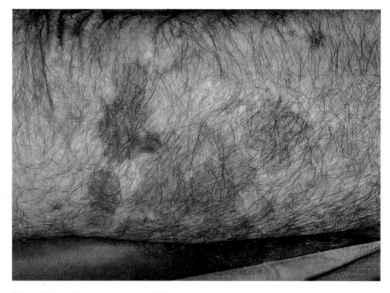

Fig. 206c Purpura – senile

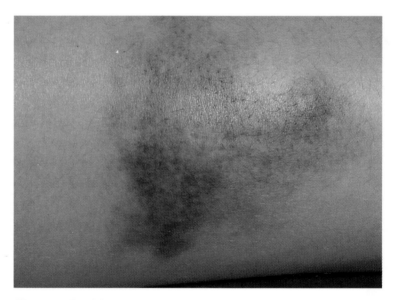

Fig. 207 Bruising

Figure 210 Pigmented
cells. They have a variety

Figure 211 Café au la
birthmarks. The findin
fibromatosis (see **Fig. 14**

Figure 207 Bruising is due to traumatic extravasation of blood. The discoloration follows a sequence of colour changes over a number of days as the blood undergoes degradation and resorption. There is sometimes a relative lack of discoloration in the centre of a large bruise at the site of impact.

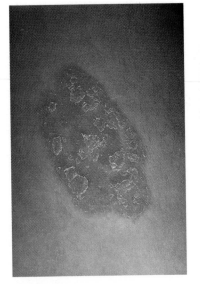

Fig. 219a Psoriasis

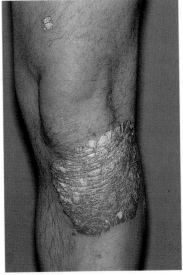

Fig. 219b Psoriasis

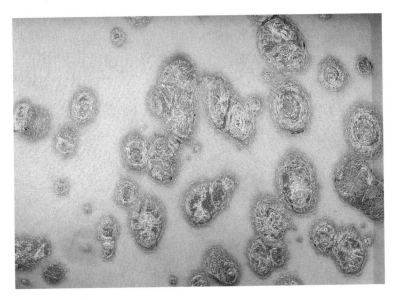

Fig. 219c Psoriasis

Figure 208 Target
shooting target. The
variety of aetiologies

Figure 209 Erythe
It is characteristic o
few hours.

Figure 219a–f Psoriasis is a common skin condition characterized by pink lesions with a scaling surface. The lesions are of various sizes and sometimes described as guttate (drop-sized) and nummular (coin-sized). Plaques of disease on extensor surfaces and on the scalp are common. There may be nail dystrophy (see **Figs 89, 90**) or pitting (see **Fig. 81**) and there is an association with arthropathy in some patients (see **Figs 99, 100a**).

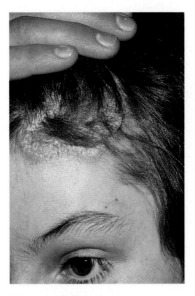

Fig. 219d Psoriasis

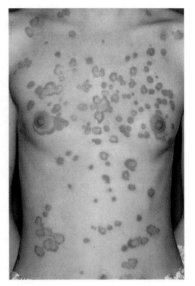

Fig. 219e Psoriasis

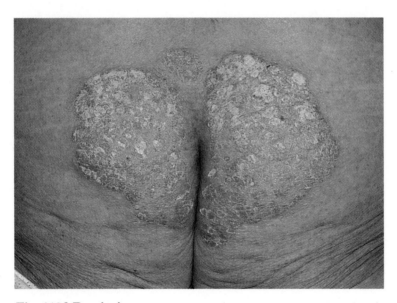

Fig. 219f Psoriasis

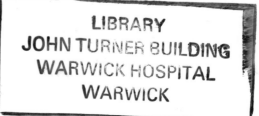

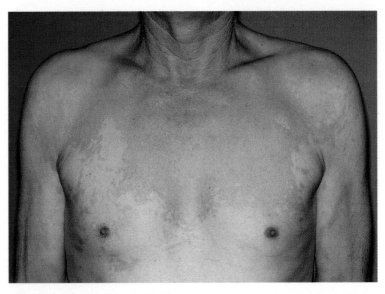

Fig. 220 Pityriasis versicolor

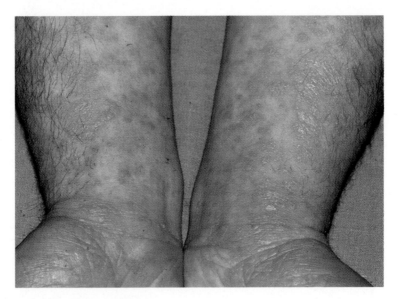

Fig. 221 Lichen planus

Figure 220 Pityriasis versicolor is due to infection with the yeast *Malessezia furfur*. There may be mild itching and scaling of the affected patches, which are typically pale on pigmented skin and darker on pale skin.

Figure 221 Lichen planus commonly occurs on the flexor aspect of the forearms and wrists and is characterized by flat-topped, violaceous, polygonal papules with whitish streaks on top.

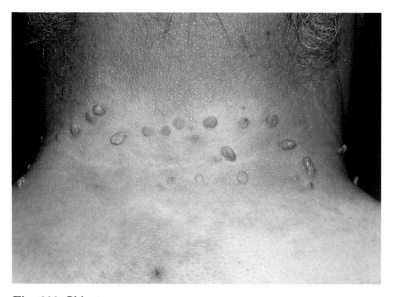

Fig. 222 Skin tags

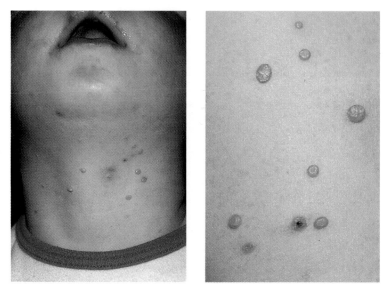

**Fig. 223a Molluscum
contagiosum**

**Fig. 223b Molluscum
contagiosum**

Figure 222 Skin tags are commonest around the neck and may be numerous. They are often polypoid, on very narrow pedicles.

Figure 223a–b Molluscum contagiosum is caused by a pox virus, which produces shiny, papular lesions often with a central pit, i.e. umbilicated.

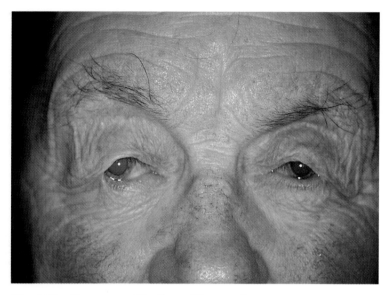

Fig. 228a Cataract – black pupillary reflex

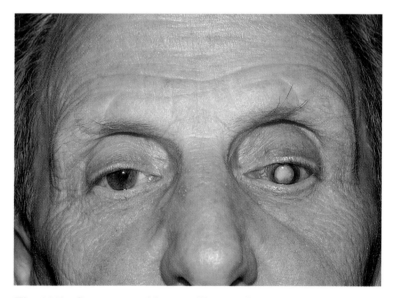

Fig. 228b Cataract – white pupillary reflex

Figure 228a–b In **Figure 228a,** the right eye shows a normal red reflex; the left reflex is absent and appears black due to the presence of cataract. In addition, the skin of both upper eyelids has lost its elasticity and drops over the eyelid margins, a condition called blepharochalasis. In **Figure 228b,** the lens of the left eye shows a dense, mature white cataract; the right red reflex is impaired due to a less-advanced cataract.

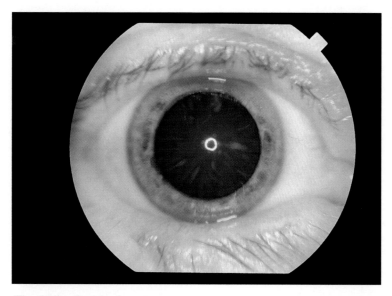

Fig. 229a Cortical cataract

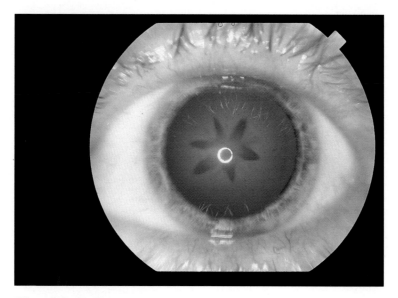

Fig. 229b Stellate cataract

Figure 229a–b Early cataract formation in the outer, cortical layers of the lens gives rise to a characteristic radial spoke pattern, similar to a bicycle wheel (**Fig. 229a**). The star-shaped cataract shown in **Figure 229b** is a typical traumatic, or concussion, cataract due to blunt trauma. These lens opacities tend not to progress or do so only very slowly.

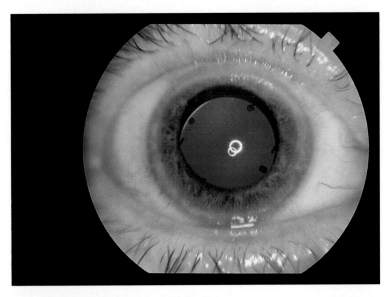

Fig. 230 Intraocular lens implant

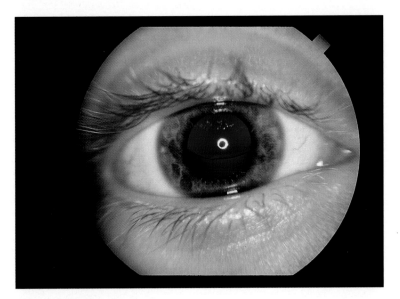

Fig. 231 Dislocated lens

Figure 230 A posterior chamber intraocular lens implant can be seen clearly in the pupil. The small round holes allow the lens to be 'dialled' into position at the time of surgery.

Figure 231 The lens has dislocated upwards, as seen by its lower pole in the pupillary axis. This pattern of dislocation, or subluxation, is typical of Marfan's syndrome. In homocystinuria, the lens characteristically dislocates downwards.

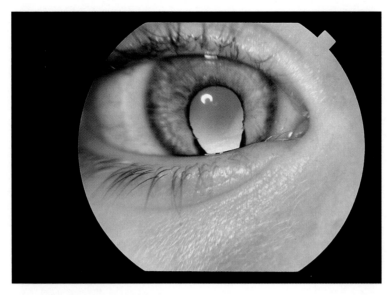

Fig. 232 Coloboma of iris

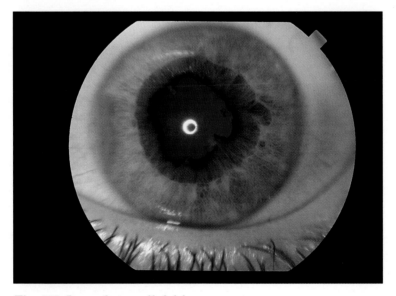

Fig. 233 Irregular pupil: iritis

Figure 232 Iris colobomata may be associated with similar defects in the choroid. The inferonasal location is typical and is due to failure of normal closure of the optic vesicle during embryonic development.

Figure 233 The pupil margin is irregular due to the presence of inflammatory adhesions to the anterior capsule of the lens, or posterior synechiae. This is a characteristic finding in most types of anterior uveitis.

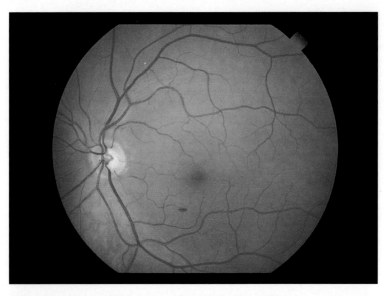

Fig. 234a Nerve fibre layer (flame) haemorrhage

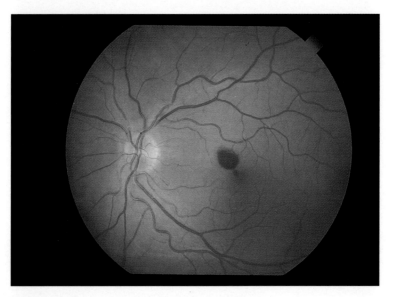

Fig. 234b Intraretinal (blot) haemorrhage

Figure 234a–b The shape of retinal haemorrhages is determined by the level of the retina in which they occur. Haemorrhage in the nerve fibre layer (**Fig. 234a**) is superficial and linear or flame shaped. Deeper retinal haemorrhages are typically round or blot shaped (**Fig. 234b**).

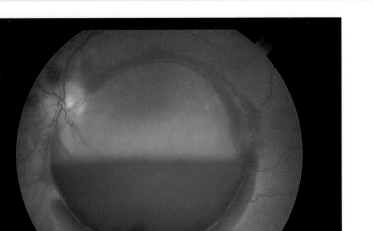

Fig. 235 Preretinal (subhyaloid) haemorrhage

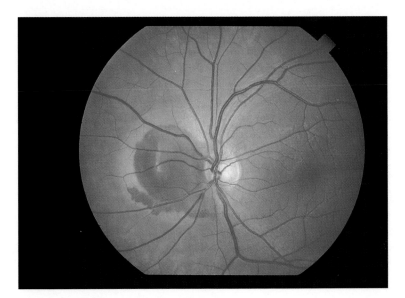

Fig. 236 Subretinal haemorrhage

Figure 235 Haemorrhage into the subhyaloid space overlying the macula may result in a localized collection of blood which has not clotted. This may settle and result in a dramatic display of the haematocrit.

Figure 236 Choroidal haemorrhage has a plum-coloured appearance, and the overlying retinal vessels can be clearly seen. This haemorrhage has resulted from blunt trauma to the eye, which has caused a localized choroidal rupture.

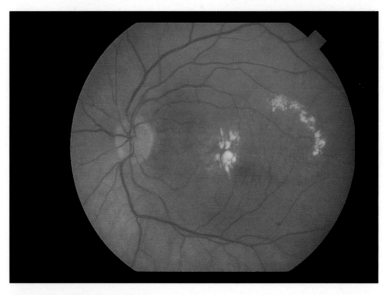

Fig. 237a Hard exudates

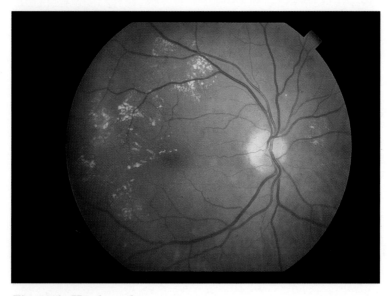

Fig. 237b Hard exudates

Figure 237a–b Hard exudates result from breakdown of the blood–retinal barrier. Macular hard exudates may be due to diabetes mellitus (**Fig 237a**). Hard exudates are sharply delineated and have a shiny, refractile appearance in comparison with cotton wool spots (**Fig. 238**) or drusen (**Fig. 239**).

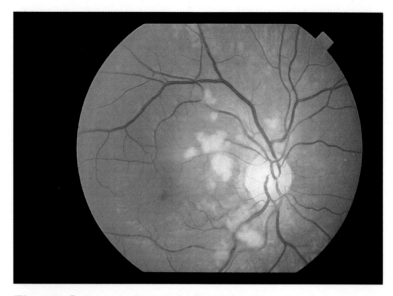

Fig. 238 Cotton wool spots (soft exudates)

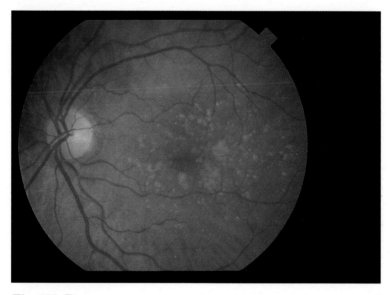

Fig. 239 Drusen

Figure 238 Cotton wool spots are microinfarcts in the nerve fibre layer of the retina. They are typically seen where this layer is thickest, around the optic disc and along the temporal vascular arcades.

Figure 239 Drusen are a common ageing change at the macula and result from degeneration at the level of Bruch's membrane, below the retinal pigment epithelium and deep to the retinal vessels. They are frequently associated with age-related macular degeneration.

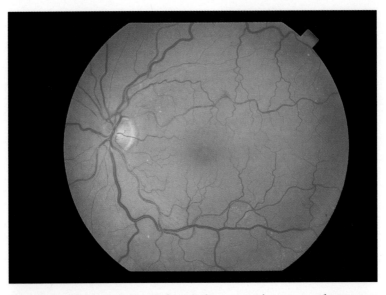

Fig. 240a Hypertensive retinopathy – arteriovenous changes

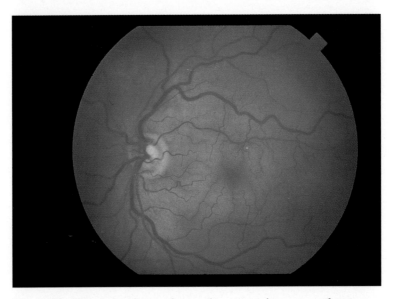

Fig. 240b Hypertensive retinopathy – arteriovenous changes

Figure 240a–b Increased vascular tortuosity and venous narrowing where the vessels cross (arteriovenous nipping or nicking) are associated with hypertension. The changes are, however, non-specific, occurring commonly in the elderly as a sign of arteriosclerosis. Venous dilatation may be seen in hypertension; hyperviscosity states may also cause this appearance, e.g. myeloma and macroglobulinaemia.

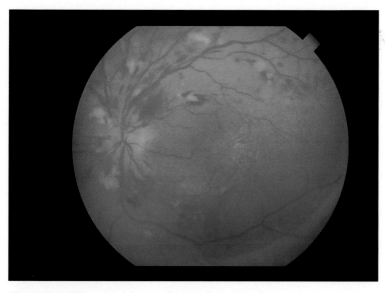

Fig. 241a Hypertensive retinopathy – accelerated hypertension

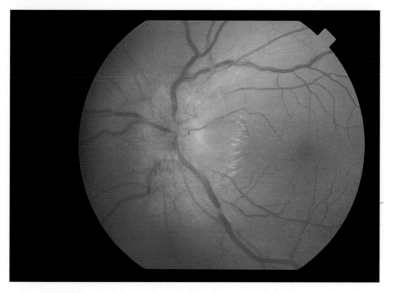

Fig. 241b Hypertensive retinopathy – accelerated hypertension

Figure 241a–b Cotton wool spots are a feature of accelerated hypertension and reflect a localized hold-up in axoplasmic transport in retinal axons due to ischaemia. A similar process can lead to optic disc swelling (papilloedema). Sustained retinal oedema has also led to fine, radial hard exudates at the macula (**Fig. 241a**) – an incomplete macular star. The optic disc may be swollen with dilated retinal veins and hard exudates between the macula and disc due to accelerated hypertension. An incomplete macular star and arteriovenous nipping (**Fig. 241b**) may be visible.

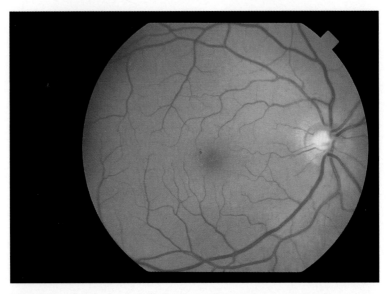

Fig. 242a Background diabetic retinopathy – minimal

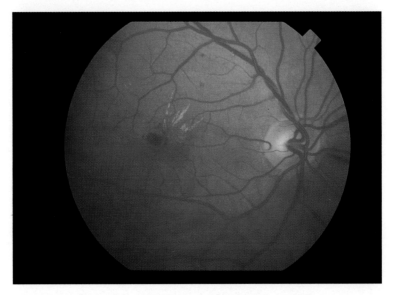

Fig. 242b Background diabetic retinopathy – mild

Figure 242a–c The characteristic features of background diabetic retinopathy are small red dots, which may be microaneurysms or small retinal haemorrhages. They may be difficult to distinguish on clinical examination (**Fig. 242a**). Retinal microaneurysms can leak plasma constituents, allowing the accumulation of lipids within the retina. This can lead to impairment of central vision if the macula is threatened (**Fig. 242b**). Leaking microaneurysms may give rise to ring-shaped, or circinate, hard exudates (**Fig. 242c**). Application of laser photocoagulation to the centre of these exudates will abolish further leakage and allow the exudates to be reabsorbed.

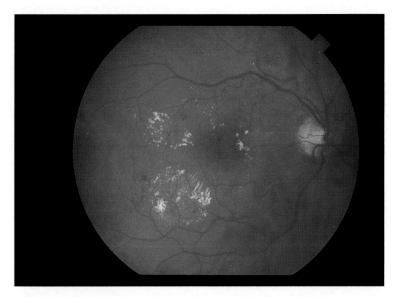

Fig. 242c Background diabetic retinopathy – moderate

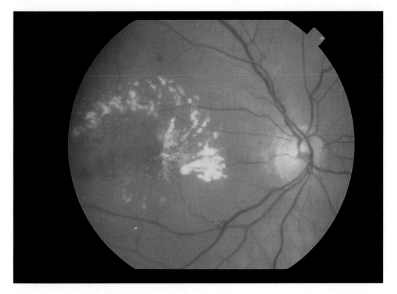

Fig. 243 Diabetic maculopathy

Figure 243 Hard exudates have accumulated at the macula and resulted in severe damage to central vision. Even if these exudates respond to laser treatment, it is unlikely that there will be much visual recovery.

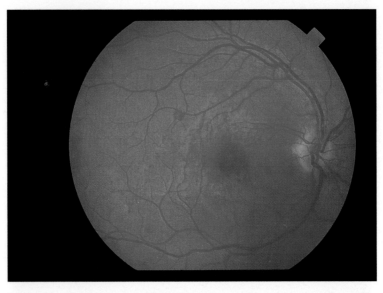

Fig. 244a Background diabetic retinopathy – 'dots' and small 'blots'

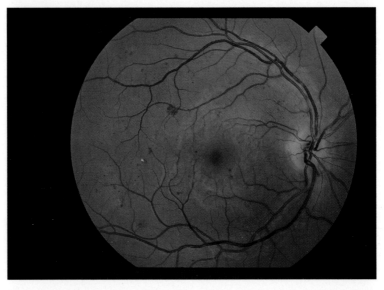

Fig. 244b Background diabetic retinopathy – red-free (green) illumination

Figure 244a–b Minimal background retinopathy consisting of microaneurysms and small haemorrhages may be difficult to detect when viewed in tungsten or halogen light (**Fig. 244a**). Use of the red-free filter to illuminate the same eye with green light allows much greater contrast and improved visualization of vascular lesions (**Fig. 244b**).

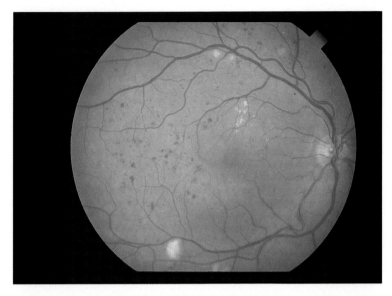

Fig. 245 Preproliferative diabetic retinopathy – cotton wool spots

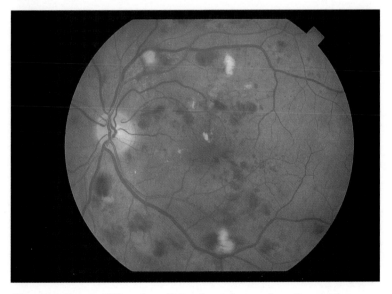

Fig. 246 Preproliferative diabetic retinopathy – large blot haemorrhages

Figure 245 Cotton wool spots, a sign of retinal infarction, indicate significant ischaemia and are considered a preproliferative feature in diabetic retinopathy. They may also be due to other causes such as accelerated hypertension.

Figure 246 Large retinal haemorrhages, greater than half a disc width in diameter, are a sign of retinal ischaemia and precede retinal neovascularization. Frequently, they are seen temporal to the macula in the watershed zone between the superior and inferior temporal vascular arcades.

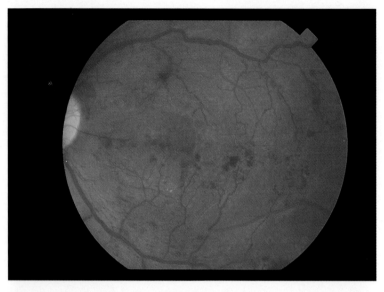

Fig. 247 Preproliferative diabetic retinopathy – beaded major vein

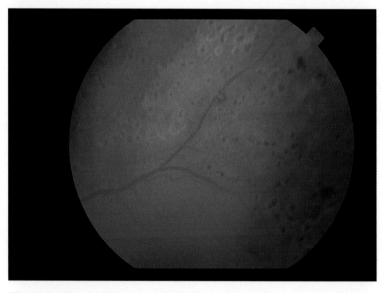

Fig. 248 Preproliferative diabetic retinopathy – venous loop (omega loop)

Figure 247 Beading of the large- and medium-sized retinal veins, as seen in the uppermost part of this example, frequently occurs in the preproliferative phase of diabetic retinopathy.

Figure 248 Other venous changes seen in preproliferative retinopathy include omega-shaped loops and reduplication (not seen in this example). This eye had laser treatment because proliferative changes ensued.

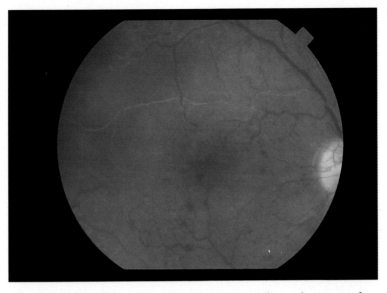

Fig. 249 **Preproliferative diabetic retinopathy – ghost vessel**

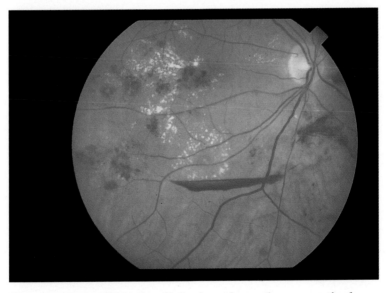

Fig. 250 **Preproliferative diabetic retinopathy – preretinal (subhyaloid) haemorrhage**

Figure 249 Arterial closure, as shown by the presence of white 'ghost' vessels, indicates retinal ischaemia in the adjacent vascular territory.

Figure 250 Blood behind the posterior vitreous face (subhyaloid or preretinal haemorrhage) settles inferiorly and outlines the site of attachment of the vitreous to the retina. The appearance has been likened to a swallow's nest. Bilateral subhyaloid haemorrhages can also occur following subarachnoid haemorrhage (Terson's syndrome).

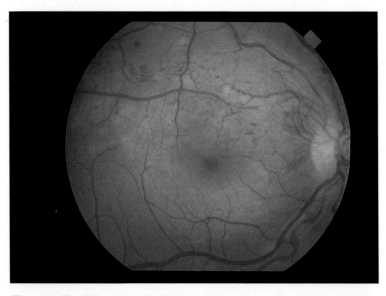

Fig. 251 Proliferative diabetic retinopathy – disc new vessels

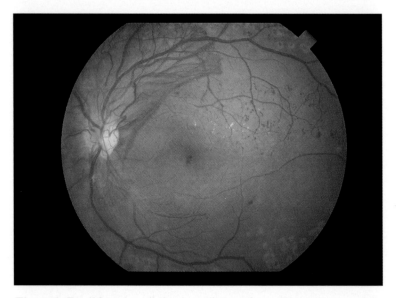

Fig. 252 Proliferative diabetic retinopathy – disc new vessels

Figure 251 Retinal new blood vessels may arise from the disc (NVD) or elsewhere (NVE). A fan of disc new vessels can be seen emanating from the superotemporal quadrant of the disc. Note the resolving cotton wool spots along the superotemporal arcade, indicative of retinal ischaemia, and the normal macula.

Figure 252 A large fan of new vessels is extending from the disc along the superotemporal arcade. Beyond the neovascular fan is a large area of ischaemic retina. In the periphery can be seen laser photocoagulation scars but further treatment is required as these new vessels are still active.

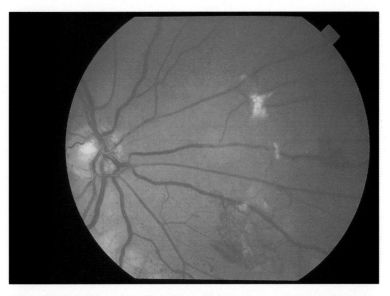

Fig. 253 Proliferative diabetic retinopathy – peripheral new vessels

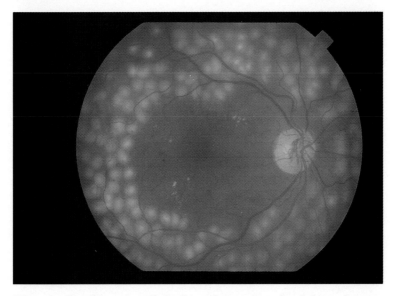

Fig. 254 Proliferative diabetic retinopathy – fresh laser burns

Figure 253 Active peripheral new vessels can be seen arising from the retinal veins. The white lesion is a neovascular complex which has regressed spontaneously leaving a gliotic scar.

Figure 254 Retinal neovascularization in diabetes is treated by panretinal ('scatter') laser photocoagulation. Fresh laser burns can be seen surrounding the macula and disc.

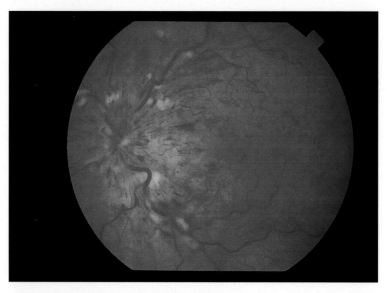

Fig. 255 Central retinal vein occlusion

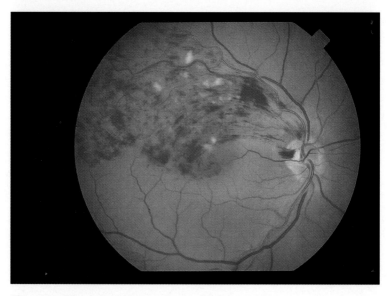

Fig. 256 Branch retinal vein occlusion

Figure 255 This shows the classical appearance of a central retinal vein occlusion with dilated retinal veins, a swollen disc and scattered haemorrhages within the retina and nerve fibre layer. In addition, there is evidence of ischaemia with the presence of cotton wool spots.

Figure 256 The superotemporal branch retinal vein has developed an occlusion; the haemorrhages extend to the fovea, indicating that visual acuity is likely to be impaired. The commonest causes of retinal vein occlusion are hypertension, diabetes and raised intraocular pressure.

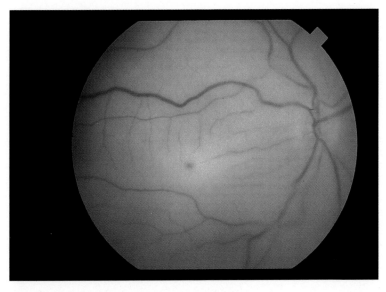

Fig. 257   Central retinal artery occlusion

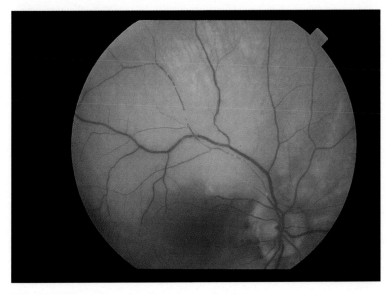

Fig. 258   Branch retinal artery occlusion

Figure 257 Occlusion of the central retinal artery results in a pale, oedematous retina. The normal blood flow through the underlying choroidal circulation produces the 'cherry-red spot' at the fovea.

Figure 258 This branch occlusion of the superotemporal retinal artery has spared the macula. The blood column in the arteries can be seen to be fragmented, a sign known as 'cattle-trucking', which occurs due to very slow blood flow.

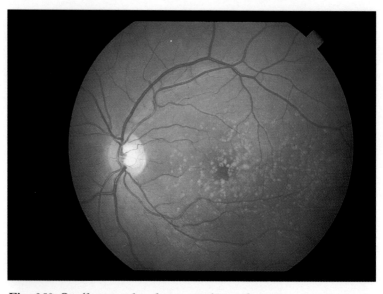

Fig. 259 Senile macular degeneration – drusen

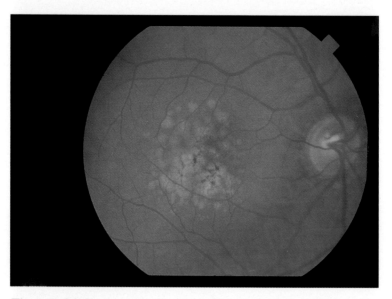

Fig. 260 Senile macular degeneration – atrophic ('dry')

Figure 259 Drusen are yellow-white bodies at the level of Bruch's membrane and are associated with age-related macular degeneration. Occasionally, they may be familial.

Figure 260 In addition to drusen, there are areas of clumping and atrophy of the retinal pigment epithelium. This is atrophic, or 'dry', age-related macular degeneration. The clinical severity of the ocular changes may be quite disproportionate to the visual impairment.

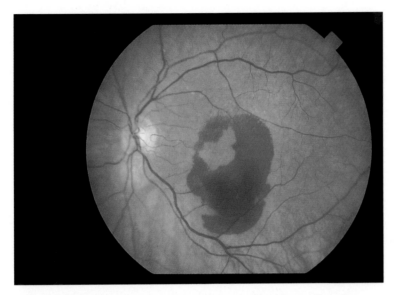

Fig. 261 Senile macular degeneration – disciform ('wet')

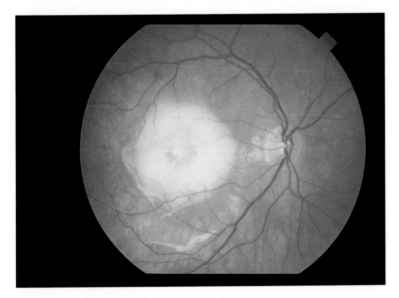

Fig. 262 Senile macular degeneration – disciform scar

Figure 261 A subretinal haemorrhage has arisen from a subretinal neovascular complex in exudative, or 'wet', age-related macular degeneration.

Figure 262 Here exudative macular degeneration has led to the development of a yellow subretinal disciform scar, which has resulted in irreversible loss of central vision.

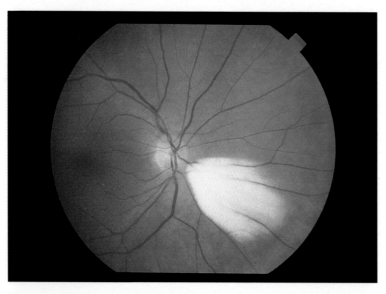

Fig. 263 Myelinated nerve fibres

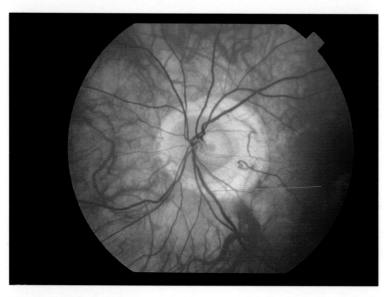

Fig. 264 Myopic disc

Figure 263 Retinal nerve fibres do not normally have a myelin sheath as this would be detrimental to visual function. An island of white myelinated fibres can be seen here obscuring the retinal vasculature near the disc.

Figure 264 In myopia, the optic disc characteristically shows a ring of choroidal atrophy. In addition, the retinal pigment epithelium is poorly pigmented and the larger choroidal vessels can clearly be seen deep to the retina.

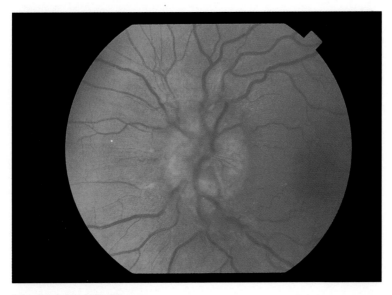

Fig. 265 Papilloedema

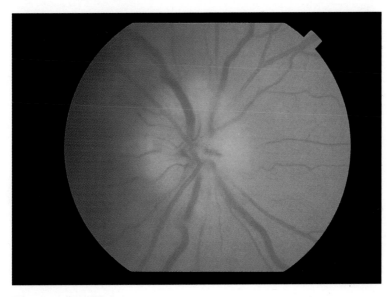

Fig. 266 Papillitis

Figure 265 In papilloedema, the optic disc is swollen with dilatation of the overlying capillaries. The normal pulsation of the retinal veins at the disc is usually lost, but visual acuity and the pupillary reflexes are normal.

Figure 266 In papillitis, the optic nerve is inflamed and ischaemic, and may appear pale and swollen with fine splinter haemorrhages. The visual acuity is usually profoundly impaired and a relative afferent pupil defect (RAPD) is likely to be present.

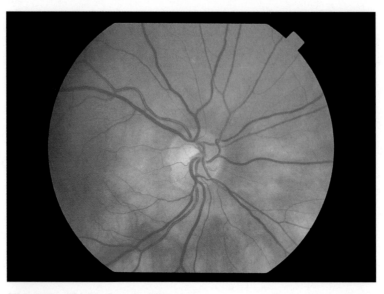

Fig. 267a Normal optic disc cup

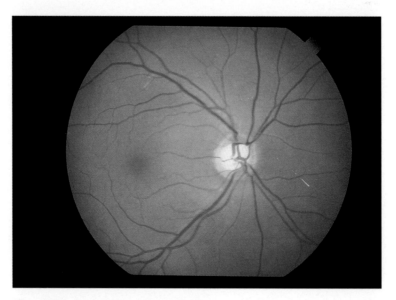

Fig. 267b Suspicious disc cupping

Figure 267a–d The normal optic disc (**Fig. 267a**) usually has a small cup that occupies about one-third of the area. The size of the cup is expressed as the decimal ratio of the vertical diameters of the cup to disc (CDR) and is around 0.3 in this eye. In **Figure 267b**, the CDR is 0.5, which is suspicious of glaucomatous disc cupping. The disc of **Figure 267c** shows gross cupping with notching of the inferior disc rim in advanced open-angle glaucoma. The whiteness of optic atrophy in **Figure 267d** compares with the more yellow colour of pathological disc cupping seen in **Figure 267c**.

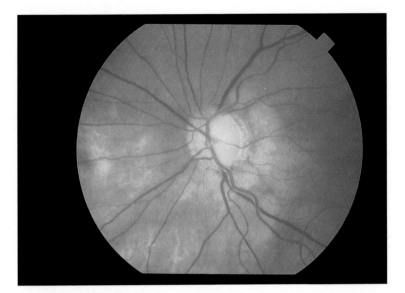

Fig. 267c Pathological disc cupping

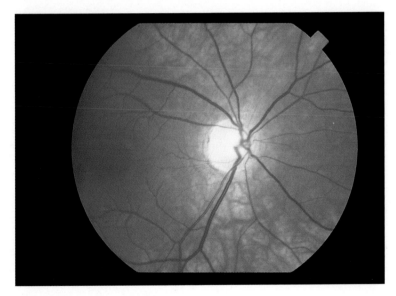

Fig. 267d Optic atrophy

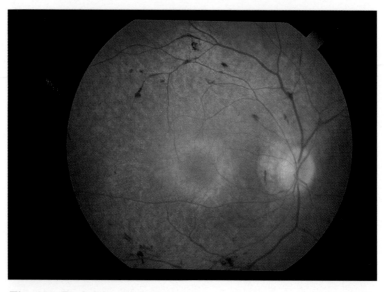

Fig. 268 Retinitis pigmentosa

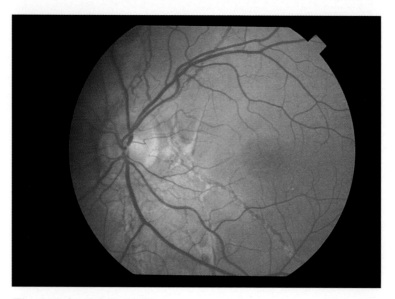

Fig. 269 Angioid streaks

Figure 268 Clumping and atrophy of the retinal pigment epithelium can be seen in the retina along the vascular arcades and in the retinal periphery, features characteristic of retinitis pigmentosa.

Figure 269 Red lines (angioid streaks) can be seen running beneath the retinal blood vessels in a radial direction out from the optic disc. There is also some subretinal scarring temporal to the disc underneath the papillomacular bundle, which has followed a choroidal rupture following blunt ocular trauma. These are the typical ocular features of pseudoxanthoma elasticum.

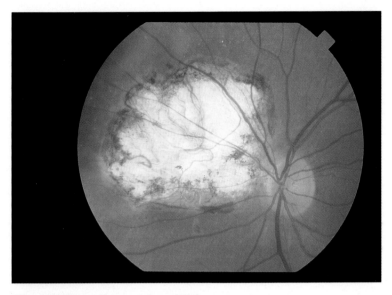

Fig. 270 Toxoplasma choroiditis

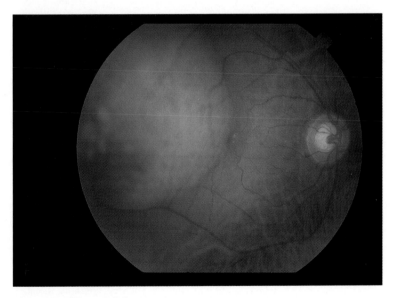

Fig. 271 Choroidal tumour

Figure 270 A large macular scar is present. There are no signs of active retinal inflammation or vitritis. The appearance is very characteristic of congenital toxoplasma infection.

Figure 271 A large elevated lesion can be seen underlying the temporal retina, extending up to the macula. These features are consistent with a choroidal tumour, most likely a primary ocular malignant melanoma.

Index